ADA POCKET GUIDE TO

bariatric
surgery

WEIGHT MANAGEMENT
DIETETIC PRACTICE GROUP

CHRISTINA K. BIESEMEIER, MS, RD, FADA,
AND JENNIFER GARLAND, MPH, RD, CDE
EDITORS

American Dietetic Association
Chicago, Illinois

Diana Faulhaber, Publisher
Elizabeth Nishiura, Production Manager

American Dietetic Association
120 South Riverside Plaza, Suite 2000
Chicago, IL 60606
www.eatright.org

10 9 8 7 6 5 4 3 2 1

Library of Congress Cataloging-in-Publication Data

ADA pocket guide to bariatric surgery / Weight Management Dietetic
Practice Group ; Christina K. Biesemeier and Jennifer Garland, editors.
    p. ; cm.
  Includes bibliographical references and index.
  ISBN 978-0-88091-424-6
  1. Obesity—Surgery—Handbooks, manuals, etc. I. Biesemeier,
Christina. II. Garland, Jennifer, 1978- III. American Dietetic
Association. Weight Management Dietetic Practice Group.
  IV. Title: Pocket guide to bariatric surgery.
  [DNLM: 1. Bariatric Surgery—rehabilitation—Handbooks. 2. Diet
Therapy—methods—Handbooks. WI 900 A191 2009]

RD540.A26 2009
617.4'3—dc22

                                                          2008042197

contents

contributors

Christina K. Biesemeier, MS, RD, FADA
Director, Clinical Nutrition Services
Vanderbilt University Medical Center
Nashville, TN
Chapters 1–6, 8

Susan Cummings, MS, RD
Clinical Programs Coordinator, MGH Weight Center
Massachusetts General Hospital
Boston, MA
Chapters 1–6 and appendixes

Jeanne Blankenship, MS, RD
Clinical Bariatric Nutrition Expert, Research Dietitian
Sacramento, CA
Chapter 9

Jennifer Garland, MPH, RD, CDE
Registered Dietitian, Diabetes Educator
Vanderbilt Eskind Diabetes Center
Nashville, TN
Chapter 8

Shelley Kirk, PhD, MS, RD
Assistant Professor of Clinical Pediatrics
Center Director, HealthWorks!
Cincinnati Children's Hospital Medical Center
Cincinnati, OH
Chapter 7

ACKNOWLEDGMENTS

The editors thank the following individuals for their assistance with Chapter 7: Kathleen B. Hrovat, MS, RD; Michelle Frank, RD; Stephen R Daniels, PhD, MD; and Thomas Inge, MD, PhD, FACS, FAAP. Thank you to Ellen Ladage, RD, CNSD, for her help with Chapter 8.

reviewers

Amy Cartwright, MS, RD
Conyngham, PA

Natalie M. Egan, MS, RD, CDE
Brigham and Women's Hospital
Boston, MA

Laura Greiman, MPH, RD
Sharp Memorial Hospital
San Diego, CA

Patti Landers, PhD, RD
Department of Nutritional Sciences
University of Oklahoma Health Sciences Center
Oklahoma City, OK

Julie Parrott, MS, RD
Plaza Medical Center of Fort Worth
Fort Worth, TX

Allison Schimmel Matson, MBA, MS, RD
Yardley, PA

Julie Schwartz, MS, RD, CSSD
Emory Bariatric Center
Atlanta, GA

Julie Walenta, MPH, RD
FirstHealth of the Carolinas
Pinehurst, NC

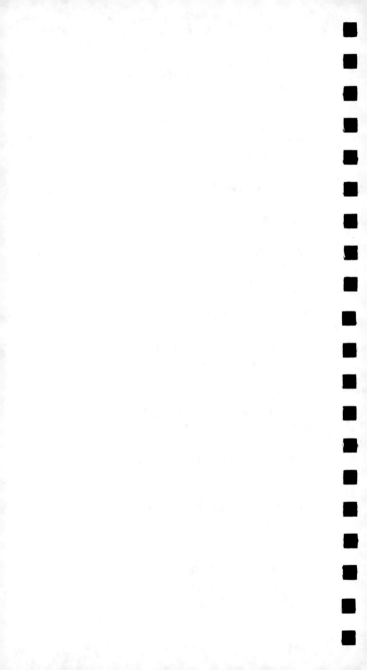

chapter 1

Weight-Loss Surgery Overview

In 2003–2004, 17% of US children and adolescents were overweight (now termed *obese*), with a body mass index (BMI) equal to or greater than the 95th percentile for their age and gender, and 32.2% of adults met criteria for obesity (BMI ≥ 30) (1). The prevalence of extreme or Class III obesity (BMI ≥ 40) during this same time period was 2.8% in men and 6.9% in women.

Comparison of National Health and Nutrition Examination Survey (NHANES) data from 1976–1980 and 2001–2002 shows that the prevalence of obesity in adults 20 to 74 years old more than doubled, from 15% to 31.3% (2). The number of individuals with extreme obesity quadrupled between 1987 and 2000. These increases— combined with the lack of effective dietary and pharmacological treatments and increasing third-party coverage of surgery—have fueled the demand for weight-loss surgery (WLS), and the number of operations performed in the United States has greatly increased.

After WLS, a large percentage of individuals with type 2 diabetes mellitus experience resolution of or significant improvement in their disease (see Table 1.1, later in this chapter). Accordingly, some in the medical field are considering WLS as a treatment for type 2 diabetes, even in people with a BMI of less than 35. This may lead to a further increase in the number of WLS procedures performed in the United States each year (3–5).

CRITERIA FOR WEIGHT LOSS SURGERY

According to the National Heart, Lung and Blood Institute (6), gastrointestinal surgery (gastric restriction or gastric bypass) can result in substantial weight loss, and therefore is a viable weight-loss option for well-informed and motivated clients with a BMI ≥ 40 as well as those with a BMI ≥ 35 who have comorbid conditions and acceptable operative risks. Before being considered for WLS, clients should also have undergone previous, non-surgical weight-loss therapies without success (6,7).

WEIGHT-LOSS SURGERY PROCEDURES

There are three categories of WLS procedures:

- **Restrictive procedures**—ie, vertical banded gastroplasty (VBG) and laparoscopic adjustable gastric banding (LAGB). With these procedures, passage of food from the upper stomach to the lower stomach is delayed. The individual feels full quickly and stops eating after small amounts of food are eaten. With LAGB, the band can be tightened to increase restriction if the client starts to feel hunger again and begins consuming increased portions of food. Nutrient deficiencies may result from restrictive procedures due to the small quantity of food consumed (8).
- **Procedures that are primarily restrictive with some malabsorption**—ie, Roux-en-Y gastric bypass (RYGBP) and vertical banded gastric bypass. With these procedures, a small gastric pouch is created at the upper end of the stomach, resulting in a substantial reduction in the storage capacity of the stomach (less than 1 ounce immediately after surgery) and a

substantial reduction in the amount of food consumed. Ingested food bypasses the entire duodenum and a short segment of the jejunum. This delays the mixing of food with bile and pancreatic enzymes, and causes mild fat and protein malabsorption. In addition, absorption of calcium, iron, and the B-complex vitamins is reduced (8).

- **Procedures that are primarily malabsorptive with some restriction**—ie, biliopancreatic diversion (BPD) and biliopancreatic diversion with duodenal switch (DS). In these procedures, approximately 60% of the small intestine is bypassed, resulting in weight loss due to malabsorption. Additional malabsorption occurs because the small intestine is rerouted, which leads to reduced mixing of food with bile and pancreatic enzymes. Deficiencies in fat-soluble vitamins (A, D, E, and K), minerals (calcium and iron), and protein can occur due to the malabsorption. With these procedures, there is some reduction in the size of the stomach, leading to a minor restrictive effect (8).

Figures 1.1, 1.2, and 1.3 illustrate types of surgeries from these three categories.

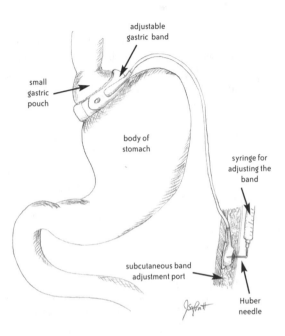

Figure 1.1 Laparoscopic adjustable gastric band (LAGB) procedure. A restrictive band is placed around the top of the stomach, reducing the capacity of the stomach. This is connected by tubing to a port into which saline is injected to perform postoperative adjustments. Reprinted with permission from Dr. Jane Pratt.

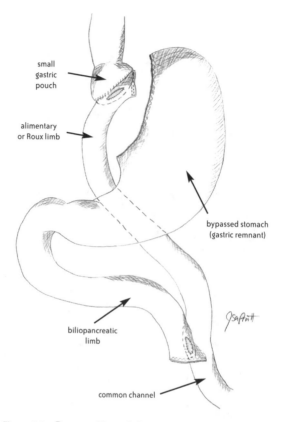

small gastric pouch

alimentary or Roux limb

bypassed stomach (gastric remnant)

biliopancreatic limb

common channel

Figure 1.2　Roux-en-Y gastric bypass procedure (RYGBP). In this procedure, a small pouch is created at the upper end of the stomach. Reprinted with permission from Dr. Jane Pratt.

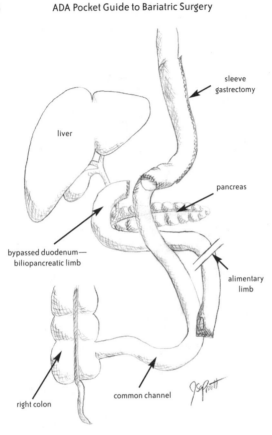

Figure 1.3 Biliopancreatic diversion (BPD) with duodenal switch. This procedure restricts the size of the stomach and bypasses approximately 60% of the small intestine. Reprinted with permission from Dr. Jane Pratt.

Most WLS procedures today are performed laparoscopically unless contraindicated. In the United States, the two most commonly performed types of WLS are RYGBP and LAGB. This pocket guide focuses on these two procedures.

WEIGHT-LOSS SURGERY OUTCOMES

Gastric Bypass

The exact mechanisms for weight loss are not known. Weight loss likely occurs due to a combination of restriction of intake and changes in neural and hormonal pathways.

According to Buchwald et al (9), in most gastric bypass studies, participants lose 60% to 70% of excess body weight (30% to 35% of total body weight) during an 18-month time period (9). In Buchwald et al's meta-analysis of 4,204 gastric bypass patients, the weighted mean loss of excess body weight was 68% (35% of total body weight) (9). (See Box 1.1 for how to calculate the percentage of excess body weight lost.) See Table 1.1 for findings regarding gastric bypass surgery and obesity comorbidities from the meta-analysis by Buchwald and associates (9).

Table 1.1　Weight-Loss Surgery and Comorbidities of Obesity: Meta-analysis Findings

	Roux-en-Y Gastric Bypass, % of Patients with Resolved Condition	Adjustable Gastric Band, % of Patients with Resolved Condition
Type 2 diabetes	84%	48%
Hyperlipidemia	93%	71%
Hypertension	75%	38%
Obstructive sleep apnea	95%	56%

Source: Data are from reference 9.

Box 1.1　Excess Body Weight Calculations

It is important to distinguish between weight loss as a percentage of excess body weight lost and weight loss as a percentage of total body weight lost. A percentage of excess weight loss is approximately twice the percentage of total body weight loss.

To determine a patient's excess body weight before weight-loss surgery:

1. Estimate what the patient's weight would be if his/her body mass index equaled 25.
2. Subtract that weight estimate from the patient's actual weight before weight-loss surgery.

To determine the percentage of excess body weight lost after weight-loss surgery:

1. Measure the amount of weight lost after surgery.
2. Divide that amount by the amount of presurgery excess body weight.
3. Multiply by 100.

Laparoscopic Adjustable Gastric Band

Weight loss occurs because the small pouch restricts volume and creates early satiety. In a meta-analysis of 1,848 individuals who had undergone gastric banding, the weighted mean weight loss was 50% of excess body weight (approximately 25% of total body weight) (9). Refer to Table 1.1 for additional data regarding obesity-related comorbidities in individual's post-LAGB (9).

PRESURGICAL ASSESSMENT

The 1991 National Institutes of Health consensus report, *Gastrointestinal Surgery for Severe Obesity,* recommends that individuals undergo careful evaluation by surgical, medical, psychiatric, and nutrition experts before being approved for surgical procedures (7). This evaluation may be performed at a surgery center that is a Center of Excellence and has a multidisciplinary team, or the surgeon may complete an evaluation first and refer clients to other team members for their individual evaluations. A Center of Excellence meets the standards of multidisciplinary care set by the American Society for Metabolic and Bariatric Surgery (ASMBS) and the American College of Surgeons (ACS).

WLS coverage by the Centers for Medicare and Medicaid Services (CMS) requires that WLS operations be performed at a Center of Excellence (10). Although insurance companies vary in their requirements for the components of the pre-WLS evaluation, the trend in the future will likely be toward increasing use of surgical centers that are designated Centers of Excellence because private insurers often follow the requirements of CMS. These standards do not require the services of a registered dietitian (RD), but most Centers of Excellence do include an RD as an integral member of the multidisciplinary team.

Surgical Evaluation

A surgical evaluation is usually completed after the client undergoes a comprehensive medical, psychological, and nutrition evaluation. However in some situations, the surgical evaluation may precede the comprehensive evaluation.

A surgical evaluation includes the following:

- Physical examination and review of past medical and surgical history
- Interview of the client by a surgeon
- Clearance for surgery
- Selection of the type of surgery and the surgical procedure (the selection is based on information and recommendations from the comprehensive medical, psychological, and nutrition evaluation)

Medical Evaluation

A complete medical evaluation for bariatric surgery includes the following:

- Physical examination including measurements (height, weight, blood pressure, pulse, respiration rate) and determination of BMI (see Box 1.2)
- Identification of medically treatable causes of obesity
- Assessment of comorbidities associated with obesity
- Laboratory tests to evaluate causes and effects of obesity; determine baseline status of glucose, hemoglobin A1C, and lipids; evaluate vitamin and mineral status; and determine the need for additional testing

- Other tests as indicated, including a sleep study, an echocardiogram (if the client took phentramine fenfloramine in the past), and evaluation of the upper gastrointestinal tract

---

Box 1.2   Tips for Measuring Weight and Height

- Use scales designed to weigh patients who weigh more than 350 lb.
- Standardize procedures for obtaining weights and heights.
- Obtain height and weight in a private setting.
- Measure height as accurately as possible; use of a wall-mounted stadiometer is recommended.

Psychological Evaluation

Clients undergo a psychological evaluation to determine their readiness for surgery and identify the following factors that may negatively or positively affect their prognosis:

- Impact of weight on daily activities and work performance
- Current psychological symptoms and stressors
- Psychosocial history: eg, psychiatric history, social and developmental functioning, family support and other support systems
- Eating patterns: eg, night eating syndrome, grazing, sweet eating
- Past and present eating disorders—eg, a high prevalence of binge eating disorder (BED) is reported in clients with obesity (11) (see Box 1.3 and Appendix H for more information on BED)
- Knowledge of risks and benefits of treatment

- Motivation
- Interpersonal consequences of weight loss (eg, client's weight affects his or her ability/willingness to establish and maintain relationships or socialize)
- Compliance with medical regimens including keeping appointments and taking medications as prescribed
- Coping mechanisms, including use of food to cope, nonfood coping mechanisms, and need to work with psychologist to develop nonfood coping mechanisms

Box 1.3   Weight-Loss Surgery in Patients with Binge Eating Disorder

Patients with BED may have somewhat poorer weight-loss maintenance outcomes after WLS, although data are limited and inconclusive. There are no randomized controlled trials comparing outcomes for patients who did and did not get pre-WLS treatment for BED. There is no strong evidence that pre-WLS treatment for BED affects short- or long-term outcomes. Pathological eating does not seem to return for at least 6 months after surgery, and may not return for much longer periods of time.

BED is *not* a contraindication to WLS.

Source: Data are from reference 12.

Nutrition Evaluation

A nutrition evaluation includes the following:

- Determination of nutritional factors that affect the client's readiness for WLS and likelihood of WLS success
- Identification of nutrient deficits
- Collection of data needed to work with the client to prepare for surgery and establish healthful lifestyle and eating habits
- Identification of nutrition-related knowledge deficits concerning WLS and setting of client education goals for both before and after WLS

ROLE OF THE REGISTERED DIETITIAN BEFORE WEIGHT-LOSS SURGERY

The RD is an important member of the multidisciplinary team who can perform the following functions:

- Lead surgical information sessions and help clients make informed decisions about WLS (12). Data indicate that pre-WLS teaching by a multidisciplinary team improves client selection and enables clients to choose the most appropriate surgical procedure, which leads to more successful outcomes (12).
- Contribute information and assessment data during the team's process of selecting clients for surgery and choosing the surgery procedure, a role supported in the *Adult Weight Management Evidence-Based Practice Guidelines* (13).
- Document the client's dieting history and anthropometric data in the letter of medical necessity for insurance approval for WLS.

- Provide the nutrition component of a pre-WLS program (see Chapter 3).

REFERENCES

1. Ogden DL, Carroll MD, Curtin LR, McDowell MA, Tabak CJ, Flegal KM. Prevalence of overweight and obesity in the United States, 1999–2004. *JAMA*. 1996;295:1549–1555.
2. Centers for Disease Control and Prevention. National Health and Nutrition Examination Survey. http://www.cdc.gov/nchs/about/major/nhanes/datalink.htm. Accessed August 29, 2007.
3. Schauer P. Metabolic surgery: the Rome Diabetes Surgery Summit and our future. Presented at the International Conference on Practical Approaches to the Treatment of Obesity 2007; Cambridge, MA.
4. Pories WJ, Swanson MS, MacDonald KG, et al. Who would have thought it? An operation proves to be the most effective therapy for adult-onset diabetes mellitus. *Ann Surg*. 1995;222:339–352.
5. Rubino F, Gagner M. Effects of obesity surgery on non-insulin-dependent diabetes mellitus. *Ann Surg*. 2002;236:554–559.
6. National Heart, Lung, and Blood Institute. *Clinical Guidelines on the Identification, Evaluation, and Treatment of Overweight and Obesity in Adults. The Evidence Report*. Bethesda, MD: National Institutes of Health; 1998. NIH publication 98–4083.
7. Gastrointestinal surgery for severe obesity. National Institutes of Health Consensus Development Conference Statement. *Am J Clin Nutr*. 1992;55(2 Suppl):615S-619S.
8. American Society for Metabolic and Bariatric Surgery. Public/Professional Education Committee—Bariatric surgery: postoperative concerns. May 23, 2007. Revised February 7, 2008. http://www.asbs.org/html/pdf/asbs_bspc.pdf. Accessed May 13, 2008.
9. Buchwald H, Avidor Y, Braunwald E, Jensen MD, Pories W, Fahrbach K, Schoelles K. Bariatric surgery: a systematic review and meta-analysis. *JAMA*. 2004;292:1724–1737.
10. Surgical Review Corporation. Bariatric Surgery Centers of Excellence: eligibility. http://www.surgicalreview.org/pcoe/tertiary/tertiary_requirements.aspx. Accessed August 29, 2007.

11. Cunningham E. What is the registered dietitian's role in the pre-operative assessment of a patient contemplating bariatric surgery? *J Am Diet Assoc*. 2006;106:153.

12. Giusti V, DeLucia A, DiVetta V, Calmes JM, Héraïef E, Gaillard RC, Burckhardt P, Suter M. Impact of preoperative teaching on surgical option of patients qualifying for bariatric surgery. *Obes Surg*. 2004;14:1241–1246.

13. American Dietetic Association Evidence Analysis Library. Adult Weight Management Evidence-Based Practice Guidelines. http://www.adaevidencelibrary.com. Accessed December 10, 2007.

FURTHER READING

Alami RS, Morton JM, Schuster R, et al. Is there a benefit to preoperative weight loss in gastric bypass patients? A prospective randomized trial. *Surg Obes Relat Dis*. 2007;3:141–145.

Alvarado R, Alami RS, Hsu G, et al. The impact of preoperative weight loss in patients undergoing laparoscopic Roux-en-Y gastric bypass. *Obes Surg*. 2005;15:1282–1286.

Boylan LM, Sugerman HJ, Driskell JA. Vitamin E, vitamin B-6, vitamin B-12, and folate status of gastric bypass surgery patients. *J Am Diet Assoc*. 1988;88:579–585.

Buffington CK, Walker B, Cowan GSM, et al. Vitamin D deficiency in the morbidly obese. *Obes Surg*. 1993;3:421–424.

Colles SL, Dixon JB, Marks P, Strauss BJ, O'Brien PE. Preoperative weight loss with a very-low-energy diet: quantitation of changes in liver and abdominal fat by serial imaging. *Am J Clin Nutr*. 2006;84:304–311.

Flancbaum L, Belsley S, Drake V, et al. Preoperative nutritional status of patients undergoing Roux-en-Y gastric bypass for morbid obesity. *J Gastrointest Surg*. 2006;10:1033–1037.

Foster GD, Makris A. Behavioral treatment: practical applications. In: Foster GD, Nonas CA, eds. *Managing Obesity: A Clinical Guide*. Chicago, IL: American Dietetic Association, 2004;76–90.

Looker AC, Dawson-Hughes B, Calvo MS, Gunter EW, Sahyoun NR. Serum 25-hydroxyvitamin D status of adolescents and adults in two seasonal subpopulations from NHANES III. *Bone*. 2002;30:771–777.

Madan AK, Orth WS, Tichansky DS, Ternovits CA. Vitamin and trace mineral levels after laparoscopic gastric bypass. *Obes Surg*. 2006;16:603–606.

Schwartz ML, Drew RL, Chazin-Caldie M. Laparoscopic Roux-en-Y gastric bypass: preoperative determinants of prolonged operative times, conversion to open gastric bypasses, and postoperative complications. *Obes Surg*. 2003;13:734–738.

Ybarra J, Sanchez-Hernandex J, Gich I, et al. Unchanged hypovitaminosis D and secondary hyperparathyroidism in morbid obesity after bariatric surgery. *Obes Surg*. 2005;15:330–335.

chapter 2

The Nutrition Care Process

The American Dietetic Association (ADA) developed the Nutrition Care Process and Model (NCPM) to achieve two goals in the 2004–2008 strategic plan (1,2):

- To increase demand and utilization of services provided by members
- To empower members to compete successfully in a rapidly changing environment

The NCPM was approved by the ADA House of Delegates in March 2003. It provides a framework and structure for the delivery of nutrition care that uses evidence-based dietetics practice and supports critical thinking and effective decision-making by the registered dietitian (RD). Use of the NCPM improves patient safety and increases the likelihood of achieving expected outcomes of nutrition care. It is intended to reduce variation in the care process, but it is not standardized care. Thus, the NCPM promotes professional autonomy and recognition of the expertise of the RD as an important member of the health care team (3,4).

It is important to note that the NCPM is to be used with ADA's *International Dietetics and Nutrition Terminology (IDNT) Reference Manual* (5). The codes that are used in the IDNT reflect term domains and a system of organizing the categories and classes within each domain and the items listed in each category or class.

PARTS OF THE NUTRITION CARE PROCESS AND MODEL

The NCPM is graphically represented by a ring diagram that includes several components (3,4):

- At the center of the model is the core: the relationship between the RD and the client.
- This core is surrounded by a circle divided into four quadrants representing the four steps of the Nutrition Care Process (NCP): nutrition assessment; nutrition diagnosis; nutrition intervention; and nutrition monitoring and evaluation. (Chapters 3 through 6 of this pocket guide will follow the four steps of the NCP. Specific information, IDNT codes, and examples will be provided for each step according to the time period before and after weight-loss surgery.)
- Wrapped around the NCP are two rings. One describes the characteristics of the RD and the other describes the characteristics of the environment in which nutrition care is provided.
- The NCP is supported by two systems: (*a*) screening and referral, by which clients gain access to nutrition care, and (*b*) outcomes management, through which data are aggregated and summarized to describe the process of care and the outcomes achieved, in order to demonstrate results and improve quality of care.

STEP 1: NUTRITION ASSESSMENT

During Step 1 of the NCP, the RD collects five different types of data (5):

- Food/nutrition-related history
- Anthropometric measurements

- Biochemical data, medical tests, and procedures
- Nutrition-focused physical findings
- Client history

Data sources include the following (5):

- Referral forms
- Client interview
- Medical records
- Physical examination and RD observation
- Team rounds
- Collaborative discussions

In completing the nutrition assessment, the RD (3,4) performs the following functions:

- Uses critical thinking skills to determine the appropriate data to collect (ie, relevant vs nonrelevant data)
- Validates collected data
- Organizes data in a meaningful way to make nutrition diagnoses
- Analyzes and interprets data, using evidence-based standards and norms for comparison (eg, the Dietary Reference Intakes or ADA's Evidence-Based Adult Weight Management Nutrition Practice Guidelines)
- Identifies nutrient requirements using reference standards and evidence-based recommendations and guidelines
- Identifies groups or clusters of abnormal or discrepant data

STEP 2: NUTRITION DIAGNOSIS

In Step 2 of the NCP, the RD identifies and labels specific nutrition problems based on the results of the nutrition assessment, the RD's clinical judgment, and the likelihood that RD interventions can resolve the nutrition diagnosis or improve its signs and symptoms (5).

Nutrition diagnoses are actual, not potential, nutrition problems. They are *not* medical diagnoses (5).

There are three nutrition diagnosis domains (5):

- Intake
- Clinical
- Behavioral/environmental

To maintain consistency in use of the IDNT, the RD reviews the client's symptoms and compares them with the signs and symptoms in the IDNT manual and then confirms the presence of at least one symptom, and preferably a cluster of symptoms, from the IDNT manual's reference sheet for the selected nutrition diagnosis (5).

After selecting the nutrition diagnosis, the RD identifies the etiology of the problem. This is important because the nutrition intervention is directed at eliminating the etiology of the nutrition diagnosis. The RD also drills down to the "root cause" etiology by identifying the most specific cause that the RD can address with a nutrition intervention (5).

The nutrition diagnosis is written in a format known as a *PES (problem, etiology, and signs/symptoms) statement* (3,4). A separate PES statement is written for each nutrition diagnosis. The PES statement includes connecting phrases to link the nutrition diagnosis to etiology ("related to") and signs and symptoms ("as evidenced by").

A client may have one or more nutrition diagnoses, depending on the complexity of his/her condition. However, both the RD and the client may find it unwieldy to focus on multiple nutrition diagnoses at one time. Therefore, nutrition diagnoses are prioritized, an activity that occurs in the next step of the NCP, nutrition intervention.

STEP 3: NUTRITION INTERVENTION

Step 3 of the NCP is defined as purposefully planned actions designed with the intent of changing a nutrition-related behavior, environmental condition, or aspect of health status. Nutrition intervention includes two components: planning and implementation.

Planning

To plan the nutrition intervention, the RD consults ADA Evidence-Based Nutrition Practice Guidelines and Toolkits and other national practice guidelines; collaborates with team members; and shares the results of the nutrition assessment and nutrition diagnoses with the client in a way that is objective and logical, yet not overwhelming or frightening.

During the planning stage, the RD and client prioritize nutrition diagnoses based on the following factors:

- Severity of the problems
- Client safety
- Client needs
- Client perceptions of the importance of the problems
- Likelihood that intervention will have a positive impact

Planning also involves working with the client to set short-term (next appointment) and long-term (entire course of nutrition intervention) goals. Examples of goals are weight loss, reduction in energy intake, behavior change, increased physical activity, and improvement in knowledge. Goals are carried out in small steps.

The RD develops a nutrition prescription that states his or her individualized recommendations for the following:

- Energy intake
- Foods
- Nutrients
- Physical activity

When setting the nutrition prescription, the RD uses critical thinking skills together with current reference standards and dietary guidelines, the client's health condition, and nutrition diagnoses. The RD links the comparative standards that were defined in the nutrition assessment step with the client's goals, via the nutrition prescription (3,4). For example, if a client's total energy requirement is 2,000 kcal/d and the goal is for the client to lose 1 pound of weight per week, the nutrition prescription for energy intake would be 1,500 kcal/d.

Planning leads to selection of specific nutrition interventions and determination of the timing and frequency of nutrition care, including follow-up appointments (3,4). IDNT defines the following four domains of interventions (5):

- Food and/or nutrient delivery
- Nutrition education
- Nutrition counseling
- Coordination of care

Examples of coordination of care include (*a*) collaboration with the surgeon and/or internist when the client is showing signs and symptoms of hypoglycemia, dehydration, or stricture; and (*b*) discussion at team meetings to provide a nutrition update to other providers on the bariatric surgery team (physician, nurse, physical therapist, etc).

Last, the RD and client define expected outcomes for each nutrition diagnosis. (Outcomes are evaluated in Step 4 of the NCP, monitoring and evaluation.)

The NCP emphasizes the client's role in the planning process. Clients are involved in choosing priority issues to address, examining the benefits and costs of different treatment strategies, and making decisions regarding which treatment strategies to implement (3,4).

Implementation

Implementation is the action phase of the nutrition intervention and involves the following (3,4):

- Ensuring that the intervention plan is carried out as intended
- Communicating the intervention plan to other team members
- Continuing data collection
- Revising the intervention plan when needed, based on the client's response and feedback

STEP 4: MONITORING AND EVALUATION

The fourth step of the NCP is monitoring and evaluation. During monitoring, the RD determines whether the intervention plan was carried out and collects new data related to the desired or expected outcomes that were selected during the planning phase of the intervention step. Evaluation includes a systematic comparison of the new data with selected criteria in order to determine progress in achieving desired or expected outcomes.

Criteria for evaluation may include the following (3,4):

- Goals
- Nutrition prescription
- Baseline status or status at a previous appointment
- Evidence-based norms and standards

Explanation of variance from expected outcomes includes:

- Observation of the impact of nutrition interventions on the etiology and signs/symptoms of the client's nutrition diagnoses
- Identification of factors that help or hinder the client's progress (eg, the RD facilitates problem-solving by the client to address or overcome identified barriers; the goals and/or intervention plan are then modified as needed to achieve desired outcomes)

The four domains defined in IDNT for monitoring and evaluation are as follows (5):

- Food/nutrition-related history outcomes
- Biochemical data, medical tests, and procedure outcomes
- Anthropometric measurement outcomes
- Nutrition-related physical finding outcomes

REFERENCES

1. American Dietetic Association Nutrition Care Process and Model. http://www.eatright.org (members-only section). Accessed May 18, 2008.

2. American Dietetic Association Strategic Plan: Mission, Vision, and Values. http://www.eatright.org (members-only section). Accessed May 18, 2008.
3. Lacey K, Pritchett E. Nutrition Care Process and Model: ADA adopts road map to quality care and outcomes management. *J Am Diet Assoc.* 2003;103:1061–1072.
4. Writing Group of the Nutrition Care Process/Standardized Language Committee. Nutrition Care Process and Model Part I: the 2008 update. *J Am Diet Assoc.* 2008; 108:1113–1117.
5. American Dietetic Association. *International Dietetics & Nutrition Terminology (IDNT) Reference Manual: Standardized Language for the Nutrition Care Process.* 2nd ed. Chicago, IL: American Dietetic Association; 2009.

chapter 3

Nutrition Care
for Presurgery Clients

This chapter describes nutrition care for clients who plan
to have weight-loss surgery (WLS). For some clients,
WLS will be scheduled in the following few weeks. Other
clients cannot have WLS until they lose an amount of
weight mandated by their insurance company or surgeon.
In some cases, WLS may be delayed 6 months or more.

The pre-WLS period, whether short or long, is a time
for the following:

- Improvement of nutritional status
- Achievement of better control of nutrition-related
  comorbidities
- Development of lifestyle and eating habits that will
  promote positive post-WLS outcomes and weight-
  loss maintenance

Nutrition management for WLS clients should use the
Nutrition Care Process (see Chapter 2) and follow the
American Dietetic Association's Adult Weight Manage-
ment Evidence-Based Practice Guidelines (1).

DESCRIPTION OF CLIENTS

The clients described in this chapter are those who have
completed the initial team evaluation, including the base-

line assessment by a registered dietitian (RD), and received initial clearance for surgery.

KEY NUTRITION ISSUES

Weight Loss Prior to Surgery

Some private insurers require clients to participate in a 3- to 6-month pre-WLS program that includes monthly documentation in the medical record of weight change as well as medical, nutrition, and/or psychological interventions. Weight loss prior to WLS may also decrease the risk of surgical complications:

- A pre-WLS weight loss of at least 5% of baseline weight has been associated with decreased operative time, a factor that may decrease surgical risk (2,3).
- In some research, liver volume was substantially decreased when participants followed a very-low-energy diet before WLS, and this was associated with a reduction in reported surgical difficulty and a decreased likelihood that a laparoscopic procedure would need to be converted to an open procedure during surgery (4).

However, findings regarding the benefits of presurgical weight loss and reduction of postoperative complications are not yet conclusive. More studies are needed to establish guidelines regarding preoperative weight loss (2,3).

Lifestyle and Behavior Changes

A reduced-calorie pre-WLS diet may acclimate the client to the post-WLS diet. Additionally, clients can initiate lifestyle and behavior changes before WLS to promote short- and long-term success after surgery. Examples of behavior changes include the following:

- Increasing structure for eating and food selection— eg, creating a daily meal plan with three meals, including breakfast, and one or two snacks; or planning ahead to ensure healthful food choices are readily available
- Reducing environmental cues to eating
- Developing awareness of hunger and satiety
- Practicing portion control
- Increasing intake of fruits, vegetables, dairy foods, whole grains, fiber, and water
- Increasing physical activity and reducing sedentary time
- Self-monitoring of eating and physical activity

Clients with binge eating disorder (BED) may benefit from pre-WLS treatment for BED, and some surgical centers require or strongly encourage behavior therapy. A reasonable course of action is to inform clients with BED that they may experience problems later that could put them at risk of weight regain and give them information about how to address those problems if they do occur.

Repletion of Vitamin and Mineral Deficits

Clients seeking WLS may have vitamin and mineral deficits. These should be identified and corrected to avoid postoperative deficiencies, the most common of which are vitamin B-12, vitamin D, folate, zinc, iron, and calcium (1,5).

Vitamin D deficiency is a major public health problem in the United States. Clients with obesity may be at higher risk for developing this deficiency than nonobese individuals (4,6,7).

Thiamin deficiency can occur in clients with obesity, with African Americans and Hispanics being at greatest risk. Symptoms include numbness and tingling in the hands and feet (6).

Refer to Appendix E and other sources, including the American Society for Metabolic and Bariatric Surgery, for recommendations for repleting specific vitamins and minerals.

Nutrition Management of Blood Glucose

Pre-WLS blood glucose control is important to reduce the risk of post-WLS infections and promote wound healing. According to the American Association of Clinical Endocrinologists, medical nutrition therapy, physical activity, oral agents, and insulin should be used as needed to optimize pre-WLS glycemic control. Targets for preoperative glycemic control are as follows (3):

- Hemoglobin A1C value of ≤ 6.5%
- Fasting blood glucose ≤ 110 mg/dL
- 1-hour postprandial blood glucose ≤ 180 mg/dL

Nutrition Education and Counseling

Clients should be counseled about the nutritional impact of the planned WLS and the post-WLS diet and supplement regimen. The RD provides the nutrition component of a pre-WLS program for clients who have been approved for WLS.

Nutrition intervention can be provided on a one-to-one basis and/or in small groups, in conjunction with pre-WLS medical and/or psychological care, such as tests, counseling, medication adjustments, and stabilization of blood

glucose. A sample outline for a pre-WLS program is provided in Appendix F.

NUTRITION ASSESSMENT

Nutrition assessment data are used to make the nutrition
diagnoses seen in the pre-WLS period. The following data
are listed in the five domains of the *International Dietetics
& Nutrition Terminology (IDNT) Reference Manual* (8).

Biochemical Data, Medical Tests, and Procedures

Data from the following should be part of the client's nutrition assessment:

- Liver function tests
- Lipid profile
- Complete blood count (CBC) with differential
- Hemoglobin A1C
- Serum iron, ferritin, and total iron-binding capacity
  (TIBC)
- Serum calcium, alkaline phosphatase
- Serum vitamin B-12
- Serum vitamin B-1 (thiamin)
- Serum folate (in women of childbearing age); con-
  sider plasma homocysteine, which is a better indica-
  tor than serum folate level of folate deficiency
- Parathyroid hormone, 25-hydroxyvitamin D
- Baseline dual-energy X-ray absorptiometry (DEXA)
  to assess bone mineral density/content especially in
  postmenopausal women

Anthropometric Measurements

The nutrition assessment should include the following anthropometric information about the client:

- Height
- Weight
- Body mass index

Nutrition-Focused Physical Findings

The following data from physical examination should be noted in the client's nutrition assessment:

- Blood pressure
- Heart rate
- Head and neck condition: eg, color and condition of gums; color and appearance of tongue; missing, damaged and/or poorly fitting teeth
- Nervous system concerns: eg, motor disturbances, including gait disturbances; diminished position sense; tingling in hands and feet
- Skin and nail condition: eg, skin lesions, pale nail beds

Food/Nutrition-Related History

Food and Nutrient Intake

The food/nutrition history should assess food and nutrient intake, including intake of the following:

- Energy
- Vitamins
- Minerals
- Protein
- Fat

- Convenience foods
- Energy-dense foods and beverages
- Alcohol

Intake patterns should also be assessed, with attention to the following:

- Meals eaten away from home
- Snacking
- Meal frequency
- Pace of eating meals
- Binge eating patterns and other disordered eating patterns: eg, night eating, grazing, sweet eating, eating large amounts when not hungry
- Eating alone

Other Issues

The nutrition assessment should also evaluate the following:

- Economic and time limitations related to the purchase or preparation of food
- Cues for eating (locations, emotions, activities, other people)
- Dieting history, including what worked and what did not and why
- Weight history and patterns of weight gain and loss
- Activity, including the types, frequency, duration, and intensity of physical activity; sedentary time (including television and computer time); and daily routines

Finally, the nutrition assessment should address aspects of the client's nutrition management, including the following:

- Knowledge and attitudes
- Weight-loss readiness and importance
- Behaviors selected to change and goals
- Confidence, readiness, and motivation to make behavior changes
- Self-monitoring abilities

Client History

As part of the nutrition assessment, RDs should investigate the types of social and family support available to clients. The assessment should note if the client seems socially isolated or connected.

Energy Requirements

The nutrition assessment should include the client's total energy expenditure. This will include the following:

- Resting metabolic rate (RMR)
- Energy requirements for physical activity

It is preferable to use indirect calorimetry to measure RMR (1). When measurement is not possible, RMR should be estimated using the Mifflin-St. Jeor equation and the client's actual body weight (1,9):

Men: RMR (kcal/d) = $10 \times$ Wt (kg) + $6.25 \times$ Ht (cm) – $5 \times$ Age (y) + 5

Women: RMR (kcal/d) = $10 \times$ Wt (kg) + $6.25 \times$ Ht (cm) – $5 \times$ Age (y) – 161

NUTRITION DIAGNOSIS

Possible Presurgery Nutrition Diagnoses

Boxes 3.1–3.10 summarize nutrition diagnoses that may be identified in the pre-WLS period, with sample etiologies and the signs and symptoms that are most likely to be present and indicative of a specific nutrition diagnosis (8).

Box 3.1   Nutrition Diagnosis: Excessive Energy Intake (NI-1.5)

Sample Etiologies
- Food- and nutrition-related knowledge deficit
- Medications that increase appetite
- Unwilling or uninterested in reducing intake

Common Signs and Symptoms
- Abnormal liver function tests after prolonged exposure (3–6 wk)
- Body fat % > 25% for men and > 32% for women
- BMI > 25 (adults)
- Weight gain
- Increased body adiposity
- Reports or observation of intake of high caloric density or large portions of food/beverages

Box 3.2   Nutrition Diagnosis: Inadequate Vitamin Intake (NI-5.9.1)

Sample Etiologies

- Lack of access to food
- Economic constraints
- Food and nutrition-related knowledge deficit
- Inappropriate food choices

Common Signs and Symptoms

- Vitamin D:
  - Ionized calcium < 3.9 mg/dL (0.98 mmol/L) with elevated parathyroid hormone, normal serum calcium, and serum phosphorus < 2.6 mg/dL (0.84 mmol/L)
  - Widening at ends of long bones
- Thiamin: erythrocyte transketolase activity > 1.20 μg/mL/h
- Vitamin B-12:
  - Serum concentration < 24.4 ng/dL (180 pmol/L)
  - Elevated homocysteine
  - Tingling and numbness in extremities
  - Diminished vibratory and position sense
  - Motor disturbances including gait disturbances
- Folic acid: serum concentration < 0.3 μg/dL (7 nmol/L); red cell folate < 315 nmol/L
- Reports or observations of:
  - Inadequate intake of foods containing vitamin as compared to requirements or recommended level (reported or observed)
  - Excessive consumption of foods that do not contain available vitamins—eg, overprocessed, overcooked, or improperly stored foods (reported or observed)
  - Prolonged use of substances known to increase vitamin requirements or reduce vitamin absorption
  - Condition associated with inadequate vitamin intake, malabsorption, or excess vitamin loss
  - Limited exposure to sunlight (vitamin D)

**Box 3.3   Nutrition Diagnosis: Inadequate Mineral Intake
            (NI-5.10.1)**

Sample Etiologies
- Lack of access to food
- Economic constraints
- Food and nutrition-related knowledge deficit
- Inappropriate food choices

Common Signs and Symptoms
- Calcium:
  - Hypocalciuria, serum 25(OH)D < 32 ng/mL
  - Diminished bone mineral density
  - Height loss
- Iron: hemoglobin < 13 g/L (2 mmol/L) (men); < 12 g/L
  (1.86 mmol/L) (women)
- Reports or observations of:
  - Insufficient mineral intake from diet compared with
    recommended intake
  - Food avoidance
  - Elimination of whole food group(s) from diet
  - Lack of interest in food
  - Inappropriate food choices
- Chronic dieting behavior
- Condition associated with inadequate mineral intake,
  malabsorption, or excess mineral loss
- Low estrogen status
- Geographic latitude and history of ultraviolet-B exposure/use
  of sunscreen
- Change in living environment/independence

Box 3.4   Nutrition Diagnosis: Altered Nutrition-Related Laboratory Value (NC-2.2)

Sample Etiologies
- Liver dysfunction
- Endocrine dysfunction
- Other organ dysfunction that leads to biochemical changes

Common Signs and Symptoms
- Abnormal liver function tests (liver disorder)
- Abnormal serum lipids
- Abnormal plasma glucose level
- Other findings of acute or chronic disorders that are abnormal and of nutritional origin or consequence
- Food and nutrition-related knowledge deficit
- Report or observation of:
  - Inadequate intake of micronutrients
  - Noncompliance with modified diet

**Box 3.5   Nutrition Diagnosis: Food and Nutrition-Related
Knowledge Deficit (NB-1.1)**

Sample Etiologies
- Harmful beliefs/attitudes about food, nutrition, and nutrition-related topics
- Lack of prior exposure to information
- Language barrier impacting ability to learn information
- Cultural barrier impacting ability to learn information
- Learning disability
- Prior exposure to incompatible information
- Prior exposure to incorrect information
- Unwilling to learn information
- Uninterested in learning information

Common Signs and Symptoms
- Verbalizes inaccurate or incomplete information
- Provides inaccurate or incomplete written response to questionnaire/written tool
- Is unable to read written tool
- No prior knowledge of need for food- and nutrition-related recommendations
- Demonstrates inability to apply food- and nutrition-related information
- Relates concerns about previous attempts to learn information
- Verbalizes unwillingness to learn information
- Verbalizes disinterest in learning information
- New medical diagnosis
- Change in existing diagnosis or condition

Box 3.6 Nutrition Diagnosis: Self-Monitoring Deficit (NB-1.4)

Sample Etiologies
- Harmful beliefs/attitudes about food, nutrition, and nutrition-related topics
- Cultural barrier impacting ability to learn information
- Learning disability
- Prior exposure to incompatible information
- Unwilling to learn information
- Uninterested in learning information
- Lack of social support to make changes
- Perception that time, interpersonal, or financial constraints prevent self monitoring
- Lack of value for behavior change
- Not ready for change
- Lack of focus and difficulty with time management

Common Signs and Symptoms
- Recorded data inconsistent with biochemical data
- Incomplete self-monitoring records
- Recorded food intake data inconsistent with weight status
- Embarrassment or anger about need for self-monitoring
- Uncertainty regarding changes that could/should be made in response to data in self-monitoring record
- No self-management equipment

**Box 3.7   Nutrition Diagnosis: Disordered Eating Pattern
            (NB-1.5)**

Sample Etiologies
- Weight preoccupation significantly influences self-esteem
- Use of food to cope with anxiety and stress
- Inability to control eating

Common Signs and Symptoms
- Food and weight preoccupation
- Fear of food
- Knowledgeable about current diet fads
- Sense of lack of control over eating
- Estimated intake of larger quantity of food in a defined time period
- Eating much more rapidly than normal, until uncomfortably full
- Consuming large amounts of food when not feeling physically hungry
- Eating alone because of embarrassment
- Feeling very guilty after overeating
- Irrational thoughts about food's effect on body
- Pattern of chronic dieting
- History of mood and anxiety disorders

Box 3.8 Nutrition Diagnosis: Limited Adherence to Nutrition-Related Recommendations (NB-1.6)

Sample Etiologies
- Harmful beliefs/attitudes about food, nutrition, and nutrition-related topics
- Unwilling to learn information
- Uninterested in learning information
- Lack of social support to make changes
- Perception that time, interpersonal or financial constraints prevent adherence
- Lack of value for behavior change
- Previous lack of success in making change
- Unsure how to meet recommendations

Common Signs and Symptoms
- Expected laboratory outcomes are not achieved
- Expected anthropometric outcomes are not achieved
- Negative body language
- Inability to recall agreed-upon changes
- Failure to complete agreed-upon homework
- Lack of compliance
- Failure to keep appointments or schedule follow-up appointments
- Uncertainty about how to consistently apply nutrition recommendations

**Box 3.9   Nutrition Diagnosis: Undesirable Food Choices
            (NB-1.7)**

Sample Etiologies
- Lack of prior exposure to or misunderstanding of
  information
- Cultural barrier impacting ability to learn information
- High level of fatigue
- Unwilling to learn information
- Uninterested in learning information
- Inadequate access to food
- Perception that time, interpersonal or financial constraints
  prevent desirable food choices
- Lack of value for behavior change
- Not ready for change
- Psychological causes such as depression or disordered eating

Common Signs and Symptoms
- Elevated lipid panel
- Findings consistent with vitamin/mineral deficit or
  deficiency
- Intake inconsistent with recommended guidelines, eg, DRIs
- Inaccurate or incomplete understanding of the guidelines
- Inability to apply guidelines
- Inability or unwillingness to select foods consistent with
  guidelines

Box 3.10   Nutrition Diagnosis: Physical Inactivity (NB-2.1)

Sample Etiologies
- Harmful beliefs/attitudes about physical activity
- Injury or lifestyle change that reduces activity
- Lack of knowledge about importance of physical activity
- Lack of social support or prior exposure to physical activity
- Perception that time, interpersonal, or financial constraints prevent desired changes
- Unwilling or uninterested in learning and/or using information
- Lack of safe environment for activity
- Lack of value for this change

Common Signs and Symptoms
- Obesity
- Excessive subcutaneous fat and low muscle mass
- Infrequency, low intensity and/or low duration of physical activity
- Large amounts of sedentary activities
- Low cardiorespiratory and/or muscle strength
- Medical diagnosis associated with or results in decreased activity
- Medications that cause somnolence and decreased cognition

Making Nutrition Diagnoses in Your Practice

To use the presurgery Nutrition Diagnoses (Boxes 3.1–3.10) and other similar material in Chapters 4, 5, and 6, review the signs and symptoms of each nutrition diagnosis listed. When working with a client, look for a cluster of the signs and symptoms listed, as they will lend strength to the diagnosis you are making. For example, for a nutrition diagnosis of Excessive Energy Intake, you might note (*a*) BMI is greater than 25, (*b*) a recent increase in body weight, and (*c*) food diary results that indicate energy consumption in excess of estimated requirements.

In terms of documentation, write the PES statement to include the client's specific data. For example:

- BMI = 35
- 45-pound weight gain in past 2 years
- Average energy intake of 2,500–3,000 kcal/d per 3-day food diary, compared with estimated requirement of 2,200 kcal/d

Use the sample etiologies in Boxes 3.1–3.10 to guide you in determining the cause of your client's nutrition diagnoses. You may also identify etiologies other than those listed.

NUTRITION INTERVENTION AND NUTRITION MONITORING AND EVALUATION

Possible Presurgery Nutrition Interventions

Boxes 3.11–3.20 list the nutrition diagnoses from Boxes 3.1–3.10 for the pre-WLS period and possible nutrition interventions for each diagnosis, with outcome indicators that can be used to evaluate the effectiveness of nutrition care. Standardized language terms are used for the interventions and indicators (8).

Box 3.11   Interventions and Outcome Indicators for Excessive Energy Intake (NI-1.5)

Possible Interventions
- Modify distribution, type, or amount of food and nutrients (ND-1.2):
  - Low-calorie or very-low-calorie diet
  - Reduced fat intake
  - Reduced carbohydrate intake
  - 4–5 meals per day, including breakfast
  - Portion control
  - Meal replacements
- Increased physical activity
- Nutrition-related medication management (prescription and/or nonprescription):
  - Initiate (ND-6.1)
  - Dose change (ND-6.2)
  - Administration schedule (ND-6.5)

Outcome Indicators
- Total energy intake (FH-1.2.1.1)—decreased by 500 kcal/d per pound of desired weight loss per week
- Types of foods/meals (FH-1.3.2.2)—number of food group servings per recommendations
- Total fat intake (FH-1.6.1.1)—reduced
- Total carbohydrate (FH-1.6.3.1)—reduced
- Self-reported adherence (FH-4.4.1)—good
- Amount of food (FH-1.3.2.1)—reduced portion sizes eaten
- Physical activity:
  - Consistency (FH-6.3.2)—increased
  - Frequency (FH-6.3.3)—increased
  - Duration (FH-6.3.4)—increased
  - Intensity (FH-6.3.6)—increased
  - Strength (FH-6.3.8)—increased
- Body mass index (AD-1.1.5)—reduced
- Weight (AD-1.1.2)—desired amount of weight loss
- Weight change (AD-1.1.4)—weight loss

Box 3.12   Interventions and Outcome Indicators for Inadequate Vitamin Intake (NI-5.9.1)

Possible Interventions
- Meals and snacks: specific foods/beverages or groups (ND-1.3)—food sources of vitamins
- Vitamin and mineral supplements (ND-3.2):
  - Multivitamin/mineral (ND-3.2.1)
  - Vitamin (specify) (ND-3.2.3)

Outcome Indicators
- Food variety (FH-1.3.2.5)—increased
- Food intake—types of food (FH-1.3.2.2)—number of food group servings of vitamin-rich foods per recommendations
- Vitamin intake (FH-1.7.1)—increased intake of specific vitamins and use of supplement per recommendations
- Self-reported adherence (FH-4.1.1)—good
- Vitamin profile (BD-1.13)—specified levels improved or within normal range

Box 3.13   Interventions and Outcome Indicators for Inadequate Mineral Intake (NI-5.10.1)

Possible Interventions
- Meals and snacks: specific foods/beverages or groups (ND-1.3)—food sources of minerals
- Vitamin and mineral supplements: multivitamin/mineral (ND-3.2.1)
- Vitamin and mineral supplements: mineral (specify) (ND-3.2.4)

Outcome Indicators
- Food variety (FH-1.3.2.5)—increased
- Food intake—types of food (FH-1.3.2.2)—number of food group servings of mineral-rich foods per recommendations
- Mineral intake (FH-1.7.2)—increased intake of specific minerals and use of supplement per recommendations
- Self-reported adherence (FH-4.1.1)—good
- Mineral profile (BD-1.9)—specified levels improved or within normal range

Box 3.14   Interventions and Outcome Indicators for Altered Nutrition-Related Laboratory Value (NC-2.2)

Possible Interventions
- Modify distribution, type, or amount of food and nutrients (ND-1.2):
  - Low-calorie or very-low-calorie diet
  - Reduced fat, cholesterol, and saturated/*trans* fat intake
  - Consistent carbohydrate intake
- Meals and snacks: specific foods/beverages or groups (ND-1.3)—food sources of carbohydrate, fat, protein, vitamins, and minerals
- Vitamin and mineral supplements: multivitamin/mineral (ND-3.2.1):
  - Vitamin (specify) (ND-3.2.3)
  - Mineral (specify) (ND-3.2.4)

Outcome Indicators
- Mineral profile (BD-1.9)—specified levels improved or within normal range
- Vitamin profile (BD-1.13)—specified levels improved or within normal range
- Glucose/endocrine profile (BD-1.5)—specific levels improved or within normal range
- Lipid profile (BD-1.7)—specific levels improved or within normal range

Box 3.15   Interventions and Outcome Indicators for Food and Nutrition-Related Knowledge Deficit (NB-1.1)

Possible Interventions
- Initial/brief nutrition education:
  - Purpose of nutrition education (E-1.1)
  - Priority modification (E-1.2)
- Comprehensive nutrition education:
  - Purpose of nutrition education (E-2.1)
  - Recommended modification (E-2.2)
  - Advanced or related topics (E-2.3)
  - Result interpretation (E-2.4)
  - Skill development (E-2.5)

Outcome Indicators
- Areas and level of knowledge (FH-3.1.1)— for specific topic areas:
  - Portion control methods
  - Use of meal replacements
  - Hunger and satiety cues
  - Nonfood coping strategies
  - Inpatient diet protocol
  - Post-WLS diet and physical activity
  - Post-WLS vitamin and mineral supplementation
  - Presurgery shopping for food and supplies

**Box 3.16   Interventions and Outcome Indicators for Self-
Monitoring Deficit (NB-1.4)**

Possible Interventions
- Nutrition counseling: theoretical basis/approach (select)
  (C-1)
- Nutrition counseling: strategies:
  ○ Motivational interviewing (C-2.1)
  ○ Goal setting (C-2.2)
  ○ Problem solving (C-2.4)

Outcome Indicators
- Ability to recall nutrition goals (FH-4.1.3)—improved
  ability; goals met
- Self-monitoring at agreed-upon rate (FH-4.1.4)—improved
  ability; reported intention to keep records; records kept and
  brought to appointment

Box 3.17   Interventions and Outcome Indicators for Disordered Eating Pattern (NB-1.5)

Possible Interventions
- Nutrition counseling: theoretical basis/approach (select) (C-1)
- Nutrition counseling: strategies:
  - Goal setting (C-2.2)
  - Self-monitoring (C-2.3)
  - Problem solving (C-2.4)
  - Social support (C-2.5)
  - Stress management (C-2.6)
  - Stimulus control (C-2.7)
  - Cognitive restructuring (C-2.8)
- Coordination of nutrition care:
  - Team meeting (RC-1.1)
  - Referral to RD with different expertise (RC-1.2)
  - Collaboration/referral to other providers (RC-1.3)

Outcome Indicators
- Self-management as agreed upon (FH-4.1.5)—improved
- Self-efficacy (FH-3.2.8)—improved
- Nutrition quality of life (FH-7.1.1):
  - Psychological factors—improved
  - Self-image—improved
  - Self-efficacy—improved
- Self-talk and cognitions (FH-3.2.9)—improved; appropriate

Box 3.18 Interventions and Outcome Indicators for Limited Adherence to Nutrition-Related Recommendations (NB-1.6)

Possible Interventions
- Interventions listed in Box 3.15
- Nutrition counseling: theoretical basis/approach (select) (C-1)
- Nutrition counseling: strategies:
  - Motivational interviewing (C-2.1)
  - Goal setting (C-2.2)
  - Problem solving (C-2.4)
  - Social support (C-2.5)
  - Stimulus control (C-2.7)
  - Cognitive restructuring (C-2.8)
  - Rewards/contingency management (C-2.10)
- Coordination of nutrition care:
  - Team meeting (RC-1.1)
  - Collaboration/referral to other providers (RC-1.3): update bariatric surgery team on factors that might impact readiness for WLS

Outcome Indicators
- Self-reported adherence (FH-4.1.1)—good
- Body mass index (AD-1.1.5)—reduced
- Weight (AD-1.1.2)—desired amount of weight loss
- Weight change (AD-1.1.4)—weight loss
- Total energy intake (FH-1.2.1.1)—decreased per nutrition prescription
- Total protein intake (FH-1.6.2.1)—amount consumed per recommendations
- Vitamin intake (FH-1.7.1)—increased intake of specific vitamins and use of supplement per recommendations
- Mineral intake (FH-1.7.2)—increased intake of specific minerals and use of supplement per recommendations
- Meal and snack pattern (FH-1.3.2.3)—improved
- Type of food/meals (FH-1.3.2.2)—improved food/meal selection
- Amount of food (FH-1.3.2.1)—reduced portion sizes

(continues next page)

Box 3.18   Interventions and Outcome Indicators for Limited Adherence to Nutrition-Related Recommendations (NB-1.6) *continued*

- Self-management as agreed upon (FH-4.1.5)—improved
- Self-monitoring at agreed-upon rate (FH-4.1.4)—improved ability; reported intention to keep records; records kept and brought to appointment
- Ability to build and use social network (FH-4.5.1)—improved; report of support systems established
- Physical activity:
  ○ Consistency (FH-6.3.2)—increased
  ○ Frequency (FH-6.3.3)—increased
  ○ Duration (FH-6.3.4)—increased
  ○ Intensity (FH-6.3.6)—increased
  ○ Strength (FH-6.3.8)—increased

Box 3.19   Interventions and Outcome Indicators for Undesirable Food Choices (NB-1.7)

Possible Interventions
- Interventions listed in Box 3.15
- Nutrition counseling: theoretical basis/approach (select) (C-1)
- Nutrition counseling: strategies:
  - Motivational interviewing (C-2.1)
  - Goal setting (C-2.2)
  - Problem solving (C-2.4)
  - Social support (C-2.5)
  - Stimulus control (C-2.7)
  - Rewards/contingency management (C-2.10)
- Coordination of nutrition care:
  - Team meeting (RC-1.1)
  - Collaboration/referral to other providers (RC-1.3)—update bariatric surgery team on factors that might impact readiness for WLS

Outcome Indicators
- Vitamin intake (FH-1.7.1)—increased intake of specific vitamins and use of supplement per recommendations
- Mineral intake (FH-1.7.2)—increased intake of specific minerals and use of supplement per recommendations
- Oral fluids amount (FH-1.3.1.1)—intake per recommendations
- Total protein intake (FH-1.6.2.1)—amount consumed per recommendations
- Total fat intake (FH-1.6.1.1)—amount and type consumed per recommendations
- Total carbohydrate intake (FH-1.6.3.1)—amount and type consumed per recommendations
- Food variety (FH-1.3.2.5)—increased; improved food/meal selection
- Type of food/meals (FH-1.3.2.2)—number of food group servings per recommendations
- Self-reported adherence (FH-4.1.1)—good

Box 3.20 Interventions and Outcome Indicators for Physical Inactivity (NB-2.1)

Possible Interventions
- Nutrition counseling: theoretical basis/approach (select) (C-1)
- Nutrition counseling: strategies:
  - Motivational interviewing (C-2.1)
  - Goal setting (C-2.2)
  - Problem solving (C-2.4)
  - Social support (C-2.5)
  - Cognitive restructuring (C-2.8)
  - Rewards/contingency management (C-2.10)
- Coordination of nutrition care: referral to community agencies/programs (RC-1.4)

Outcome Indicators
- Physical activity:
  - Consistency (FH-6.3.2)—increased
  - Frequency (FH-6.3.3)—increased
  - Duration (FH-6.3.4)—increased
  - Intensity (FH-6.3.6)—increased
  - Strength (FH-6.3.8)—increased
- Self-monitoring at agreed-upon rate (FH-4.1.4)—improved ability; reported intention to keep records; records kept and brought to appointment
- Self-reported adherence (FH-4.1.1)—good

Nutrition Interventions and Outcomes in Your Practice

To use Boxes 3.11–3.20 and other similar boxes in Chapters 4, 5, and 6, find the boxes for the nutrition diagnoses you have made. Consider the intervention strategies that are listed for each diagnosis. As necessary to provide effective nutrition intervention, expand on these strategies and define them in more depth. Select one or more of the outcome indicators listed for the nutrition diagnosis to evaluate at the next client appointment or contact. Define the outcome indicators, so that you will know if they are achieved or not. For example:

- Total energy intake (FI-1.1.1) = 1,500 kcal/d
- Physical activity:
  - Consistency/frequency (BE-4.3.1)—Increased = Walking at slow to moderate pace three times per week
  - Duration (BE-4.3.1)—Increased = 10–15 minute walking bouts

PRESURGERY CASE STUDY

Refer to Box 3.21 for an example of how the Nutrition Care Process might be applied to a client before WLS.

**Box 3.21   Nutrition Care Process Case Study
             for Presurgery Period**

Nutrition Diagnosis (PES Statement): Excessive energy
intake related to undesirable food choices of sugar-sweetened
beverages as evidenced by intake history of six regular sodas
per day

Nutrition Prescription: Weight reduction diet (~ 1,400 to
1,500 kcal/d); increase physical activity to light activity;
reduction in sugar-sweetened beverages

Nutrition Intervention: Modify distribution, type, and
amount of foods and nutrients within meals or at specified
time. Nutrition counseling: Transtheoretical stages of change;
motivational interviewing to clarify benefits vs cost of
changing; cognitive behavioral theory; problem solving to
identify ways to increase physical activity and find substitutes
for sugar-sweetened beverages. Coordination of nutrition care:
referral to community program for walking.

Nutrition Monitoring and Evaluation: At follow-up
appointment in 2 weeks, the quantity of sugar-sweetened
sodas, amount of physical activity, and selection of healthful
food/meals will be monitored and evaluated.

REFERENCES

1. American Dietetic Association Evidence Analysis Library: Adult
   Weight Management Evidence-Based Practice Guidelines.
   http://www.adaevidencelibrary.com. Accessed December 10,
   2007.
2. Ybarra J, Sanchez-Hernandex J, Gich I, et al. Unchanged
   hypovitaminosis D and secondary hyperparathyroidism in morbid obesity after bariatric surgery. *Obes Surg*. 2005;15:330–335.
3. Mechanick JI, Kushner RF, Sugerman HJ, for the writing group.
   Executive summary of the recommendations of the American
   Association of Clinical Endocrinologists, the Obesity Society,
   and American Society for Metabolic & Bariatric Surgery med-

ical guidelines for clinical practice for the perioperative nutritional, metabolic, and nonsurgical support of the bariatric surgery patient. *Endocr Pract.* 2008;14:318–336.

4. Looker AC, Dawson-Hughes B, Calvo MS, Gunter EW, Sahyoun NR. Serum 25-hydroxyvitamin D status of adolescents and adults in two seasonal subpopulations from NHANES III. *Bone.* 2002;30:771–777.

5. Foster GD, Markis A. Behavioral treatment: practical applications. In: Foster GD, Nonas CA, eds. *Managing Obesity: A Clinical Guide.* Chicago, IL: American Dietetic Association; 2004:76–90.

6. Madan AK, Whitney SO, Tichansky DS, Ternovits CA. Vitamin and trace mineral levels after laparoscopic gastric bypass. *Obes Surg.* 2006;16:603–606.

7. Buffington CK, Walker B, Cowan GSM, et al. Vitamin D deficiency in the morbidly obese. *Obes Surg.* 1993;3:421–424.

8. American Dietetic Association. *International Dietetics & Nutrition Terminology (IDNT) Reference Manual: Standardized Language for the Nutrition Care Process.* 2nd ed. Chicago, IL: American Dietetic Association; 2009.

9. Mifflin MD, St. Jeor ST, Hill LA, Scott BJ, Daugherty SA, Koh YO. A new predictive equation for resting energy expenditure in healthy individuals. *Am J Clin Nutr.* 1990;51:241–247.

chapter 4

Nutrition Care in the Immediate Postsurgery Period

This chapter focuses on the postoperative nutrition care of weight-loss surgery (WLS) clients from surgery until 2 months postsurgery.

DESCRIPTION OF CLIENTS

The clients described in this chapter are those who have had WLS without complications and been discharged to home after a short hospital stay. The typical length of stay in the hospital after WLS varies among facilities and depends on the type of surgery performed.

KEY NUTRITION ISSUES

Advancement of Diet

A systematic review by an American Dietetic Association Evidence Analysis Work Group determined that there is no evidence to support any specific protocol of post-WLS diet stages (1). Until there is evidence, facilities can develop their own diet protocols or use one from another facility that has performed a large number of surgeries.

The diet advancement protocols for Roux-en-Y gastric bypass (RYGBP) and laparoscopic adjustable gastric banding (LAGB) in Appendixes B and C are examples of diet stages. In these protocols, stages I through III are used in the immediate postsurgery time period.

Diet Stage I

The first stage in the diet advancement protocol is a very short-term, clear liquid diet that is used in hospitals on post-WLS days 1 and 2. (Refer to Appendixes B and C.)

Diet Stage II

The second stage in the protocol is a full liquid diet started at home after discharge and continued until the next appointment with the surgeon and/or registered dietitian (RD), which occurs 10 and 14 days after WLS. (Refer to Appendixes B and C.) Clients with LAGB may experience hunger while on the full liquid diet.

Diet Stage III: Texture Progression

In the sample protocols provided in Appendixes B and C, this stage has three steps:

- Step 1 is initiated 10 to 14 days after WLS and used for 1 week (Box 4.1).
- Step 2 is initiated at 3 weeks after WLS and used for 1 week.
- Step 3 is initiated at 4 weeks after WLS and used until the client is seen by a RD for follow-up.

Box 4.1 Sample Meal Plan for Laparoscopic Adjustable Gastric Banding Diet Stage III, Week 1

Note: Advance to this diet 10 to 14 days after surgery.

Upon waking: Slowly sip 4–8 oz water or clear liquid to hydrate.

Breakfast: 8 oz protein shake, sipped very slowly, **or** two eggs[a]
Sip at least 8 oz clear liquids between breakfast and lunch.

Lunch: 6–8 oz yogurt **or** 8 oz protein drink
Sip at least 8 oz clear liquids between lunch and afternoon snack. Take two chewable children's "complete" multivitamins.

Afternoon snack: 4 oz sugar-free pudding **or** 1 cup nonfat (skim) or 1% milk
Sip 8 oz clear liquids before dinner.

Dinner: 8 oz protein shake **or** condensed tomato soup made with milk
Take one calcium chew or 1 tablespoon liquid calcium.
Sip 4–8 oz clear liquids between dinner and evening snack.

Evening snack: 4 oz yogurt **or** 4 oz cottage cheese[b] **or** ½ cup egg salad[a]
Take one calcium chew or 1 tablespoon liquid calcium.

---

[a]Eggs should be very moist, such as soft poached eggs or scrambled eggs. If making egg salad, use a low-fat mayonnaise. Dice eggs into tiny pieces, use a baby fork to eat, and chew, chew, chew.
[b]Choose *low-fat* cottage cheese, no chunks of fruit, blended only.
Reprinted with permission from Sue Cummings, MS, RD.

Hydration Status

A client may be dehydrated if he or she is constipated and is not on drugs that cause constipation. If dehydration is suspected, assess fluid intake.

Protein Status

To minimize loss of lean body mass, WLS clients must consume sufficient protein. Clients should be encouraged to limit starchy carbohydrates and eat high-quality protein foods along with soft fruits and well-cooked vegetables at every meal and snack (2).

Tolerance to Food

Food intolerances are common in the period immediately following WLS. Clients may also have altered taste and changes in food preferences.

Regurgitation without nausea or true vomiting is common when clients eat or drink too much food, eat or drink too rapidly, or do not chew food thoroughly. Consistent reminders to eat and drink slowly and use mindful eating exercises are helpful.

Clients may report that food gets "stuck." This may be more commonly experienced when food is poorly chewed and when eating dry meats, chicken, other dense proteins, and some starches.

Diarrhea

Diarrhea can occur after RYGBP. It may be due to undigested food passing rapidly through the gastrointestinal tract or caused by previously undiagnosed lactose intolerance. Diarrhea is not an adverse effect associated with LAGB.

Hypometabolism

Hypometabolism is common during the first few months following WLS and leads to cold intolerance and fatigue. These symptoms usually subside within 6 to 9 months, when the rate of weight loss decreases and energy intake increases (2).

NUTRITION ASSESSMENT

At the client's first appointment with an RD after WLS, which typically occurs 2 to 6 weeks after WLS (timing varies among facilities), the RD completes a reassessment. This involves collecting, recording, measuring, and assessing the following data from the client, the medical record, and other providers (see Figure F.1 in Appendix F).

Biochemical Data, Medical Tests, and Procedures

Data from the following should be part of the client's nutrition assessment:

- Complete blood count (CBC) with differential
- Hemoglobin A1C, if last value > 1 month prior to appointment
- Blood urea nitrogen (BUN)
- Other data as indicated

Anthropometric Measurements

The nutrition assessment should include the following anthropometric information about the client:

- Weight
- Body mass index
- Amount and rate of weight change

Nutrition-Focused Physical Findings

The following data from the physical examination should be noted in the client's nutrition assessment:

- Blood pressure
- Heart rate
- Condition of skin and mucous membranes (eg, dry skin does not readily return to position after pinching)
- Observation of confusion, concentration changes, motor/gait disturbances, dizziness, and/or decreased position sense
- Understanding of diet stages and guidelines
- Amount, type, and duration of physical activity
- Client concerns

Food/Nutrition-Related History

Food and Nutrient Intake

The RD should assess the client's intake of the following:

- Fluid
- Vitamin/mineral supplements (see Appendix D for supplementation information)
- Protein
- Energy-dense beverages

The food and nutrition history should also note inappropriate food choices or inappropriate food consistency and whether eating patterns indicate excessive food intake in a defined time period.

Food Tolerance

The following issues related to tolerance of food should be assessed:

- Changes in taste preferences and tolerance of food
- Difficulty swallowing
- Hunger
- Thirst
- Lactose intolerance

Other Issues

Additional factors to evaluate in the food and nutrition history include the following:

- Emotional distress surrounding mealtime
- Ability to purchase and prepare foods
- Ability to adhere to diet guidelines
- Ability to keep self-monitoring logs

Client History

The RD should assess client reports of the following:

- Diarrhea and/or constipation and/or vomiting
- Decreased urination
- Confusion, concentration changes, motor/gait disturbances, dizziness, and/or decreased position sense
- Fatigue
- Changes in medications, including changes in types taken, doses, or the administration schedule
- Medical/health history—changes in comorbidities or their treatment
- Schedule of appointments with surgeon, primary care physician, and other team members

NUTRITION DIAGNOSIS

Some nutrition diagnoses, etiologies, signs, and symptoms in the period following WLS may be the same as those from the period before surgery. These diagnoses include the following (3):

- Self-monitoring deficit
- Limited adherence to nutrition-related recommendations
- Food and nutrition-related knowledge deficit
- Physical inactivity

Refer to Chapter 3 for the etiologies, signs, and symptoms to use when writing problem, etiology, signs/symptoms (PES) statements for these diagnoses.

Other nutrition diagnoses may be the same as those used during the presurgery period, but they will have different etiologies and/or signs and symptoms from those noted before WLS. Refer to Boxes 4.2–4.4 (3).

**Box 4.2   Nutrition Diagnosis: Inadequate Vitamin Intake
(NI-5.9.1)**

Sample Etiologies
- Not taking vitamin supplement
- Vitamin supplement lacks one or more recommended vitamins

Common Signs and Symptoms
- Reports not taking supplement or taking supplement without all recommended vitamins

Note: New nutrition laboratory tests are generally not obtained until 8 to 12 weeks after weight-loss surgery.

**Box 4.3   Nutrition Diagnosis: Inadequate Mineral Intake
(NI-5.10.1)**

Sample Etiologies
- Not taking mineral supplement
- Mineral supplement lacks one or more recommended minerals
- Use of calcium carbonate instead of calcium citrate

Common Signs and Symptoms
- Reports not taking supplement
- Reports taking supplement without all recommended minerals

Note: New nutrition laboratory tests are generally not obtained until 8 to 12 weeks after weight-loss surgery.

Box 4.4   Nutrition Diagnosis: Undesirable Food Choices (NB-1.7)

Sample Etiologies
- Unwillingness to select foods consistent with guidelines
- Lack of or change in support systems
- Lack of motivation to adhere to guidelines

Common Signs and Symptoms
- Inability, unwillingness, or disinterest in selecting food consistent with guidelines:
  - Reports consuming solid foods
  - Reports consuming caffeine
  - Reports lack of interest or willingness to follow guidelines

Boxes 4.5 to 4.9 list nutrition diagnoses seen for the first time in the immediate period following WLS, with sample etiologies, and the most likely signs and symptoms (3). Box 4.10 provides examples of PES statements.

Box 4.5   Nutrition Diagnosis: Excessive Oral Food/Beverage Intake (NI-2.2)

Sample Etiologies
- Unwilling to reduce or uninterested in reducing intake
- Food and nutrition-related knowledge deficit: Laparoscopic adjustable gastric banding clients may be unaware that the band may not be "filled" until their first postoperative surgical visit, which may be 4 to 8 weeks after band placement or longer. Although there may be swelling at the band placement site, there is no restriction until the band is filled.

Common Signs and Symptoms
- Weight gain not attributed to fluid retention
- Report of intake of:
  ○ Foods/beverages with high calorie-density
  ○ Large portions of food/beverages
  ○ Amounts that exceed estimated needs
- Binge eating patterns

Box 4.6   Nutrition Diagnosis: Inadequate Protein Intake (NI-5.7.1)

Sample Etiologies
- Difficulty consuming enough protein due to volume limitations
- Lack of access to food
- Economic constraints
- Food and nutrition-related knowledge deficit
- Inappropriate food choices
- Lack of suppression of gut hormones due to type of procedure (LAGB)

Common Signs and Symptoms
- Estimated intake of protein insufficient to meet requirements:
  ○ Report of being physically unable to consume enough to meet requirements
  ○ Not using protein supplement
- Reports of excessive hunger with LAGB

Box 4.7   Nutrition Diagnosis: Inadequate Fluid Intake (NI-3.1)

Sample Etiologies
- Inappropriate food choices
- Food and nutrition-related knowledge deficit

Common Signs and Symptoms
- Elevated blood urea nitrogen or serum sodium
- Dry skin and mucous membranes, poor skin turgor
- Urine output < 30 mL/hr
- Report of:
  - Consuming < 48 oz total fluid daily
  - Thirst
  - Difficulty swallowing
  - Diarrhea

Box 4.8   Nutrition Diagnosis: Swallowing Difficulty (NC-1.1)

Sample Etiologies
- Insufficient chewing of food
- Eating too much food
- Eating too rapidly
- Eating tough foods, doughy bread, overcooked and dry meat (steak, chicken)
- Stricture

Common Signs and Symptoms
- Feeling of "food getting stuck"
- Pain while swallowing
- Regurgitation

Box 4.9 Nutrition Diagnosis: Altered GI Function (NC-1.4)

Sample Etiologies
- Anastamosis stricture
- Compromised GI tract function
- Inability to digest lactose
- Rapid emptying of sugars and carbohydrates from gastric pouch into the small intestine, triggering a release of gut peptides
- Antibiotic use

Common Signs and Symptoms
- Nausea, vomiting, diarrhea, gas, abdominal cramping and/or pain
- Constipation
- Avoidance of specific foods/food groups due to GI symptoms
- Onset of symptoms associated with the ingestion of simple sugars, lactose, and/or fried foods

Box 4.10   Sample Diagnosis (PES) Statements for the Immediate Post-WLS Period

---

Diagnosis: Self-monitoring deficit (NB-1.4)
Self-monitoring deficit related to lack of awareness of the importance of self-monitoring, as evidenced by self report of not keeping food and physical activity logs

Diagnosis: Inadequate vitamin and mineral (calcium) intake (NI-5.9.1 and NI-5.10.1)
Inadequate vitamin and mineral (calcium) intake related to not taking vitamin and calcium supplements, as evidenced by self report of stopping supplements due to their bad taste

Diagnosis: Altered GI function (NC-1.4)
Altered GI function related to consumption of milk and apparent lactose intolerance, as evidenced by gas and explosive diarrhea after milk ingestion

---

NUTRITION INTERVENTION AND NUTRITION MONITORING AND EVALUATION

Boxes 4.11–4.17 list new nutrition diagnoses for the immediate time period following WLS, with possible nutrition interventions and outcome indicators (3). The outcome indicators can be used to evaluate the effectiveness of the interventions in the Monitoring and Evaluation step of the Nutrition Care Process.

Box 4.11   Interventions and Outcome Indicators for Inadequate Fluid Intake (NI-3.1)

Possible Interventions
- Meals and snacks: specific foods/beverages or groups (ND-1.3)—attention to consumption of fluids per guidelines for diet stage

Outcome Indicators
- Oral fluid amounts (FH-1.3.1.1)—amount consumed follows diet stage guidelines
- Urine volume (BD-1.12.5)—desired mL/24 hr
- Skin turgor (PD-1.1.8)—normal
- Gastrointestinal tract (PD-1.1.5)—mucous membrane appearance normal

Box 4.12   Interventions and Outcome Indicators for Swallowing Difficulty (NC-1.1)

Possible Interventions
- Meals and snacks:
  - Modify type and amount of foods eaten at meals and snacks (ND-1.2)—attention to consumption of quantities per guidelines for diet stage
  - Other (ND-1.4): Eat slowly; set utensil down between swallowed bites
- Coordination of nutrition care:
  - Team meeting (RC-1.1): communicate all problems identified and planned or recommended interventions to physician and bariatric surgery team
  - Collaboration/referral to other providers (RC-1.3)—including speech pathologist as needed

Outcome Indicators
- Amount of food (FH-1.3.2.1)—selection of quantity of foods at meals and snacks per recommendations
- Nutrition-focused physical findings: gastrointestinal tract (PD-1.1.5)—reduction or elimination of reports of difficulty swallowing

Box 4.13   Interventions and Outcome Indicators for Altered GI Function (NC-1.4): All Types

Possible Interventions

Nutrition Education

Note: Select intervention based on amount of teaching needed.

- Initial/brief nutrition education: purpose of nutrition education (E-1.1)
- Initial/brief nutrition education: priority modification (E-1.2)
- Comprehensive nutrition education: purpose of nutrition education (E-2.1)
- Comprehensive nutrition education: recommended modification (E-2.2)
- Comprehensive nutrition education: advanced or related topics (E-2.3)

Coordination of Nutrition Care

- Team meeting (RC-1.1): communicate all problems identified as well as planned or recommended interventions to physician and bariatric surgery team
- Collaboration/referral to other providers (RC-1.3)

Outcome Indicators

- Food and nutrition knowledge: areas and level of knowledge (FH-3.1.1)—increased for specific topic areas
- Type of food/meals (FH-1.3.2.2)—selection of foods at meals and snacks per recommendations
- Self-reported adherence (FH-4.1.1)—reports of food selection indicates adherence to modifications

Box 4.14   Interventions and Outcome Indicators for Altered GI Function (NC-1.4): Dumping Syndrome[a]

Possible Interventions

- Meals and snacks: modify *type* of foods eaten at meals and snacks to limit/omit (ND-1.2):
  - Lactose
  - Refined sugars
  - High–glycemic index carbohydrates
  - Fats
  - Fried foods
- Modify *distribution* of foods and fluids at meals and snacks (ND-1.2)—ie, foods and fluids are not consumed at the same time.

Outcome Indicators

- Nutrition-focused physical findings: digestive system (PD-1.1.5)—reduction or elimination of reports of dumping syndrome

---

[a]See Box 4.13 for additional interventions and outcome indicators (those applicable to all types of altered GI function).

Box 4.15   Interventions and Outcome Indicators for Altered GI Function (NC-1.4): Antibiotic-Associated Diarrhea or *Clostridium difficile* Colitis[a]

Possible Interventions
- Meals and snacks: modify type of foods eaten at meals and snacks (ND-1.2)—omit lactose
- Nutrition-related medication management: initiate (ND-6.1)—recommend consideration of initiation of medication to control diarrhea
- Bioactive substance supplement: initiate (ND-3.3.1)—recommend initiation of probiotics to restore GI tract flora

Outcome Indicators
- Bioactive substance intake (FH-1.5.2)—intake of probiotics per recommendations
- Nutrition-focused physical findings: digestive system (PD-1.1.5)—reduction or elimination of reports of diarrhea

[a]See Box 4.13 for additional interventions and outcome indicators (those applicable to all types of altered GI function).

Box 4.16   Interventions and Outcome Indicators for Altered GI Function (NC-1.4): Constipation[a]

Possible Interventions
- Meals and snacks: specific foods/beverages or groups (ND-1.3)—attention to consumption of fluids per guidelines for diet stage
- Bioactive substance supplement:
  - Initiate (ND-3.3.1)—recommend initiation of fiber supplement
  - Discontinue (ND-3.3.6)—discontinue caffeine per guidelines

Outcome Indicators
- Oral fluid amounts (FH-1.3.1.1)—amount consumed per diet stage guidelines
- Fiber intake (FH-1.6.4)—intake of fiber per recommendations
- Total caffeine intake (FH-1.5.3.1)—omission of intake of caffeine per recommendations
- Nutrition-focused physical findings: digestive system (PD-1.1.5)—reduction or elimination of reports of constipation

[a]See Box 4.13 for additional interventions and outcome indicators (those applicable to all types of altered GI function).

Box 4.17   Interventions and Outcome Indicators for Altered GI Function (NC-1.4): Malabsorption[a]

Possible Interventions
- Meals and snacks: specific foods/beverages or groups (ND-1.3)—attention to consumption of protein per guidelines for diet stage
- Vitamin and mineral supplements:
  - Vitamins (ND-3.2.3)—vitamin B-complex and vitamin B-12
  - Minerals (ND-3.2.4)—calcium (citrated form) and iron (take with vitamin C)

Outcome Indicators
- Total protein intake (FH-1.6.2.1)—intake of protein per recommendations
- Vitamin intake (FH-1.7.1)—intake of specified vitamins per recommendations; use of supplements
- Mineral intake (FH-1.7.2)—intake of specified minerals per recommendations; use of supplements

[a]See Box 4.13 for additional interventions and outcome indicators (those applicable to all types of altered GI function).

CASE STUDY OF THE IMMEDIATE
POST-WLS TIME PERIOD

Refer to Box 4.18 for an example of how the Nutrition Care Process might be applied to a client immediately after WLS.

Box 4.18 **Nutrition Care Process Case Study for the Immediate Postsurgery Period**

Client had laparoscopic adjustable gastric banding (LAGB) and is on full liquids. She comes to a follow-up appointment complaining of hunger and reporting intake of a limited amount of protein.

Nutrition Diagnosis: Inadequate protein intake related to inappropriate food choices, as evidenced by report of consuming foods with low protein content

Goals
- Protein intake per recommendations
- Decreased hunger

Nutrition Prescription: 60–80 g protein per day

Interventions
Food and/or Nutrient Delivery
- Meals and snacks: modify type of food (ND-1.2)—modify meals and snacks to include soft, solid protein foods:[a]
  - To prevent or reduce excessive hunger and increase protein intake, start by replacing one full liquid meal with soft, solid protein foods such as eggs and cottage cheese.
  - Increase intake of soft, solid protein foods over next 1 to 2 weeks.
  - Continue to advance diet texture in subsequent weeks.

Nutrition Education
- Purpose of nutrition education (E-1.1)
- Priority modifications (E-1.2)

Monitoring and Evaluation
- Evaluate protein intake and reports of hunger.

[a]Use of very high-protein powders and supplements may cause dehydration. Refer to Box 4.1 for sample meal plan.

REFERENCES

1. American Dietetic Association Evidence Analysis Library. Nutrition Care in Bariatric Surgery. http://www.adaevidence library.com. Accessed December 10, 2007.
2. Mechanick JI, Kushner RF, Sugerman HJ, for the writing group. Executive summary of the recommendations of the American Association of Clinical Endocrinologists, the Obesity Society, and American Society for Metabolic & Bariatric Surgery medical guidelines for clinical practice for the perioperative nutritional, metabolic, and nonsurgical support of the bariatric surgery patient. *Endocr Pract.* 2008;14:318–336.
3. American Dietetic Association. *International Dietetics & Nutrition Terminology (IDNT) Reference Manual: Standardized Language for the Nutrition Care Process.* 2nd ed. Chicago, IL: American Dietetic Association; 2009.

chapter 5

Nutrition Care of Clients 2 Months to 2 Years After Surgery

This chapter covers the time period from 2 months after weight-loss surgery (WLS) to 2 years post-WLS. There are two distinct phases in this time period: (*a*) 2 to 6 months post-WLS, and (*b*) 6 months to 2 years post-WLS.

RATE OF WEIGHT LOSS

In this period, the rate of weight loss is generally slower than the rapid rate of loss seen earlier. Rates will vary among clients. Weight loss often occurs in stages, with periods of loss followed by weight plateaus. (Clients can track their progress by keeping a weight-loss graph.)

Clients with laparoscopic adjustable gastric banding (LAGB) generally lose about 1 to 3 pounds per week. This rate of weight loss is slower than the typical rate for clients who have had Roux-en-Y gastric bypass (RYGBP). Factors that may influence the rate of weight loss among LAGB clients include their pre-LAGB weight, height, gender, abdominal fat distribution, and physical activity, as well as their food choices.

CHANGES IN HEALTH STATUS

During the 2 years following WLS, many obesity-related comorbid conditions may be resolved or improved. For example:

- Clients with type 2 diabetes may achieve normal blood glucose levels or have substantially improved blood glucose control (1). Achievement of normal blood glucose levels is more prevalent following RYGBP than with LAGB (2).
- Mild to moderate sleep apnea may be completely resolved. Clients with more severe sleep apnea may continue to have residual apneic episodes (3–5).
- Hypoventilation may be reduced, because intra-abdominal pressure decreases as visceral fat is lost.

Within 6 months of WLS, serum lipid levels may improve, with reductions in total cholesterol and triglyceride levels. High-density lipoprotein (HDL) cholesterol levels gradually increase, with significant improvements by 12 months post-WLS (6).

The following conditions may also improve during the first 2 years after WLS:

- Urinary incontinence
- Gastroesophageal reflux
- Systemic hypertension
- Venous stasis disease
- Obesity-related cardiomyopathy and cardiac function
- Disordered sleep
- Degenerative joint disease and mobility
- Non-alcoholic steatorrhea hepatitis (NASH)

- Asthma
- Polycystic ovary syndrome
- Infertility

KEY NUTRITION ISSUES

Hydration Status

If a client is constipated and is not on drugs that may cause constipation, he or she may be mildly to severely dehydrated. Assess fluid intake if dehydration is suspected.

Protein Status

To avoid excessive loss of lean body mass, clients must consume sufficient protein. Encourage clients to increase protein intake to approximately 60 to 80 g/d. Excessive protein intake should be avoided.

Clients vary in their tolerance of protein. If clients are not well hydrated, excessive protein intake contributes to dehydration.

At 3 to 5 months post-WLS, RYGB clients may lose hair, which can be very distressing. Hair loss may be due to reduced protein or B vitamin intake, or it may be caused by hormonal changes related to fat loss.

Vitamin and Mineral Status

Compliance with recommendations for supplementation is important.

Advancement of Diet

In this time period, the diet texture advances from soft, moist, pureed, ground, or diced protein foods to more solid protein foods, along with fruits, vegetables, and whole grain starches. Texture advances and food tolerance vary among clients. Discourage clients from comparing their own progress with that of other clients.

Lifestyle and Behavior Changes

During this period, clients must adopt and adhere to self-management practices. For example, they need to eat slowly and chew food thoroughly. Also, because they can tolerate larger amounts of food than they did immediately after surgery, clients must pay attention to the amount of food eaten and their energy balance.

Registered dietitians (RDs) should help clients adhere to nutrition-related recommendations and understand their importance. Clients should also be encouraged to increase their physical activity and participate in structured exercise programs.

Hunger

Hunger is a concern for some clients. It has been theorized that a negative energy balance during weight loss stimulates the production of ghrelin, a gastrointestinal hormone. This is an adaptive mechanism that increases appetite.

The type of WLS seems to affect clients' feelings of hunger:

- Hunger initially decreases after RYGBP. It is theorized that this happens because ghrelin production is markedly suppressed after this procedure (7).
- After LAGB, clients experience hunger, which may be caused by a weight loss–induced increase in ghrelin production (8). One study found that ghrelin levels were increased at 6 and 12 months after surgery, and then subsequently returned to normal levels for weight (6). This may explain why this procedure is associated with smaller amounts of excess weight loss compared with RYGBP (7,8).

MONITORING AND POST-WLS FILLS/BAND ADJUSTMENTS FOR LAGB

The first fill usually occurs 4 to 8 weeks after band placement. After the band is filled for the first time, there is a slow diffusion of fluid from the band, which decreases restriction over time. Clients need to have their weight loss and hunger assessed to determine when subsequent band fills, referred to as *band adjustments*, should occur (see Box 5.1).

Box 5.1   Laparoscopic Adjustable Gastric Banding (LAGB) Band Assessment

---

Symptoms of a Band That Is Too Tight
- Dysphagia
- Nighttime cough
- Heartburn/reflux/vomiting

Symptoms of a Band That Is Too Loose
- Increased portion sizes
- Hunger between meals
- Good tolerance of food despite poor eating style ("I can eat anything")
- Poor weight loss

During the first year following WLS, LAGB clients are typically seen by the team at the surgical center every 4 to 6 weeks for monitoring, education, and support and to assess need for a band adjustment (refer to Appendix F for sample assessment forms). The frequency of visits varies among surgery centers.

Clients reach an optimal stable adjustment level. After this point, they no longer need regular fills/adjustments. This generally occurs 1 to 3 years after band placement.

However, as long as the band is in place, all LAGB clients should be seen by the team at the surgical center at least once a year for monitoring of weight and nutritional status and comorbidity assessment.

NUTRITION ASSESSMENT

At each post-WLS appointment, the RD collects and evaluates a similar set of data. Refer to the assessment section of Chapter 4 for a list of data and to Appendix F for examples of post-WLS assessment forms. Additional data to collect at each visit during this time period are described in the following sections.

Food/Nutrition-Related History

In each assessment, the RD should note the following about the client's intake patterns:

- Meal and snack frequency
- Level of hunger before meals
- Level of fullness after meals
- Amount of food client is able to eat at one sitting
- Excessive intake of food in a defined time period
- Meals eaten away from home
- Duration of meals
- Consumption of liquids at same time as solids

Nutrition-focused Physical Findings

The assessment should include client reports of the following:

- Nausea, heartburn, reflux, or dysphagia
- Nighttime cough

- Abdominal pain and cramping
- Stomach grumbling

NUTRITION DIAGNOSIS

Many nutrition diagnoses and PES statements for the 6 months to 2 years following WLS are the same as those described in Chapter 4 for the immediate post-WLS period. These diagnoses include the following (9):

- Inadequate protein intake
- Inadequate vitamin intake
- Inadequate mineral intake
- Inadequate fluid intake
- Altered GI function
- Self-monitoring deficit
- Limited adherence to nutrition-related recommendations
- Undesirable food choices
- Food and nutrition-related knowledge deficit
- Physical inactivity

Refer to Chapter 4 for possible etiologies and signs and symptoms to use when writing problem, etiology, signs/symptoms (PES) statements for these diagnoses. Other nutrition diagnoses (Boxes 5.2–5.4) can reflect new problems that may occur 6 months to 2 years after WLS (9). Box 5.5 provides examples of PES statements.

**Box 5.2   Nutrition Diagnosis: Excessive Oral Food/Beverage
            Intake (NI-2.2)**

Possible Etiologies
- In Roux-en-Y gastric bypass (RYGBP) clients:
  - Increased absorption of food, especially fat, as
    gastrointestinal tract adapts over time
  - Enlargement of the gastric pouch over time
  - Anastomotic dilatation
- In laparoscopic adjustable gastric banding (LAGB) clients:
  - Widening of stoma due to weight loss or not getting fills

Common Signs and Symptoms
- Weight plateau
- Intake that exceeds estimated or measured energy needs:
  - Report of increased meal/snack frequency
  - Report of grazing

Box 5.3   Nutrition Diagnosis: Swallowing Difficulty (NC-1.1)

Possible Etiologies
- Adverse effect of restrictive bypass procedure caused by:
  - Rapid intake
  - Inadequate chewing
  - Intake of large pieces of food

Common Signs and Symptoms
- Pain while swallowing
- Feeling of food "getting stuck":
  - Report of heartburn or backing up of food into esophagus
  - Chest pressure
  - Tightness in throat

Box 5.4   Nutrition Diagnosis: Disordered Eating Pattern (NB-1.5)

Possible Etiologies
- Weight preoccupation substantially influences self-esteem
- Use of food to cope with anxiety and stress
- Inability to control eating
- Return of eating disorder

Common Signs and Symptoms
- Food and weight preoccupation
- Fear of food
- Sense of lack of control over eating
- Eating much more rapidly than normal, until feeling uncomfortably full
- Consuming large amounts of food when not feeling physically hungry
- Eating alone because of embarrassment
- Feeling very guilty after overeating
- Irrational thoughts about food's effect on body
- Report of starving during day and binge eating at night
- History of mood and anxiety disorders
- History of binge eating; report of starving during day and binge eating at night

Box 5.5   Sample Diagnosis (PES) Statements for 6 Months to 2 Years Following Weight-Loss Surgery

---

Diagnosis: Inadequate fluid intake (NI-3.1)
Inadequate fluid intake related to not drinking between meals, as evidenced by report of thirst and two to three episodes of orthostatic hypotension per week.

Diagnosis: Inadequate vitamin and mineral (calcium) intake (NI-5.9.1 and NI-5.10.1)
- Roux-en-Y gastric bypass (RYGBP) client: Inadequate vitamin and mineral (calcium) intake related to not taking vitamin and calcium supplements, as evidenced by altered nutrition related labs, high PTH, and low vitamin D levels
- Laparoscopic adjustable gastric banding (LAGB) client: Inadequate vitamin intake related to not taking vitamin supplements, as evidenced by low serum folate level

Diagnosis: Altered GI function (NC-1.4)
- Altered GI function related to consumption of milk and apparent lactose intolerance, as evidenced by gas and explosive diarrhea after milk ingestion
- Altered GI function related to eating too fast, as evidenced by vomiting after eating

Diagnosis: swallowing difficulty (NC-1.1)
- Swallowing difficulty related to eating large pieces of food without chewing properly, as evidenced by pain in mid-chest and sensation of food being "stuck"

NUTRITION INTERVENTION AND NUTRITION MONITORING AND EVALUATION

Boxes 5.6–5.11 list possible nutrition interventions and outcome indicators for nutrition diagnoses made in the 6 months to 2 years following WLS (9). The outcome indicators can be used to evaluate the effectiveness of the interventions in the monitoring and evaluation step of the Nutrition Care Process.

Box 5.6   Interventions and Outcome Indicators for Inadequate Fluid Intake (NI-3.1)

Possible Interventions
- Meals and snacks: specific foods/beverages or groups (ND-1.3)—attention to consumption of fluids per guidelines for diet stage

Outcome Indicators
- Oral fluid amounts (FH-1.3.1.1)—amount consumed per diet stage guidelines
- Urine volume (BD-1.12.5)—desired mL/24 hr
- Skin turgor (PD-1.1,8)—normal
- Digestive system (PD-1.1.5)—mucous membrane appearance normal

Box 5.7   Interventions and Outcome Indicators for Altered GI Function (NC-1.4): All Types

---

Possible Interventions

Nutrition Education Interventions

Note: Select interventions based on the amount of teaching needed.

- Initial/brief nutrition education: purpose of nutrition education (E-1.1)
- Initial/brief nutrition education: priority modification (E-1.2)
- Comprehensive nutrition education: purpose of nutrition education (E-2.1)
- Comprehensive nutrition education: recommended modification (E-2.2)
- Comprehensive nutrition education: advanced or related topics (E-2.3)

Coordination of Nutrition Care Interventions

- Team meeting (RC-1.1): communicate all problems identified as well as planned or recommended interventions to physician and bariatric surgery team.
- Collaboration/referral to other providers (RC-1.3)

Outcome Indicators

- Type of food/meals (FH-1.3.2.2)—food/meal selection per recommendations
- Self-reported adherence (FH-4.1.1)—reports of food selection indicate adherence to modifications
- Food and nutrition knowledge: areas and level of knowledge (FH-3.1.1)— for specific topic areas

Box 5.8   Interventions and Outcome Indicators for Altered GI Function (NC-1.4): Dumping Syndrome[a]

Possible Interventions
- Meals and snacks: modify *type* of foods eaten at meals and snacks (ND-1.2)—limit/omit:
  - Lactose
  - Refined sugars
  - High–glycemic index carbohydrates
  - Fats
  - Fried foods
- Meals and snacks: modify *distribution* of foods and fluids at meals and snacks (ND-1.2)—ie, foods and fluids should not be consumed at the same time

Outcome Indicators
- Nutrition-focused physical findings: digestive system (PD-1.1.5)—Reduction or elimination of reports of dumping syndrome

[a]See Box 5.7 for additional interventions and outcome indicators (those applicable to all types of altered GI function).

Box 5.9 Interventions and Outcome Indicators for Altered GI Function (NC-1.4): Constipation[a]

Possible Interventions
- Meals and snacks: specific foods/beverages or groups (ND-1.3):
  - Attention to consumption of fluids per guidelines for diet stage
  - Increased intake of dietary fiber from fruits, vegetables, and whole grains
- Initiate bioactive substance supplement (ND-3.3.1)—recommend initiation of fiber supplement
- Discontinue bioactive substance supplement (ND-3.3.6)—discontinue caffeine

Outcome Indicators
- Oral fluid amounts (FH-1.3.1.1)—amount consumed per diet stage guidelines
- Fiber intake (FH-1.6.4)—intake of fiber per recommendations
- Total caffeine intake (FH-1.5.3.1)—omission of intake of caffeine per recommendations
- Nutrition-focused physical findings: digestive system (PD-1.1.5)—Reduction or elimination of reports of constipation

[a]See Box 5.7 for additional interventions and outcome indicators (those applicable to all types of altered GI function).

Box 5.10   Interventions and Outcome Indicators for Altered GI Function (NC-1.4): Malabsorption[a]

Possible Interventions
- Meals and snacks: specific foods/beverages or groups (ND-1.3)—Attention to consumption of protein per guidelines for diet stage.
- Vitamin supplements (ND-3.2.3)—B-complex vitamins and vitamin B-12
- Mineral supplements (ND-3.2.4)—calcium (citrated form) and iron (take with vitamin C)

Outcome Indicators
- Total protein intake (FH-1.6.2.1)—intake of protein per recommendations
- Vitamin intake (FH-1.7.1)—intake of specified vitamins per recommendations; use of supplements
- Mineral intake (FH-1.7.2)—intake of specified minerals per recommendations; use of supplements

[a]See Box 5.7 for additional interventions and outcome indicators (those applicable to all types of altered GI function).

**Box 5.11   Interventions and Outcome Indicators for
Undesirable Food Choices (NB-1.7)**

Possible Interventions

Nutrition Education Interventions

Note: Select intervention based on amount of education
needed.

- Initial/brief nutrition education: purpose of nutrition
  education (E-1.1)
- Initial/brief nutrition education: priority modification (E-1.2)
- Comprehensive nutrition education: purpose of nutrition
  education (E-2.1)
- Comprehensive nutrition education: recommended
  modification (E-2.2)
- Comprehensive nutrition education: advanced or related
  topics (E-2.3)

Coordination of Care Interventions

- Team meeting (RC-1.1): communicate all problems
  identified as well as planned or recommended interventions
  to physician and bariatric surgery team
- Collaboration/referral to other providers (RC-1.3)

Outcome Indicators

- Food intake:
  - Amount of food (FH-1.3.2.1)—selection of quantity of
    foods at meals and snacks per recommendations
  - Type of food/meals (FH-1.3.2.2)—selection per
    recommendations
  - Meal/snack pattern (FH-1.3.2.3)—selection per
    recommendations
- Food and nutrition knowledge: areas and level of knowledge
  (FH-3.1.1)—increased for specific topic areas

CASE STUDIES

Refer to Boxes 5.12 and 5.13 for examples of how the Nutrition Care Process might be applied to clients in the 2 years following WLS.

Box 5.12   Nutrition Care Process Case Study: A Discouraged Client

---

Client comes for a follow-up appointment. His weight loss is less than what was noted at previous appointments, and he says he is discouraged by slowing of weight loss.

Nutrition Diagnosis: Food and nutrition-related knowledge deficit related to unrealistic expectations about the pattern of post–weight-loss surgery (WLS) weight loss, as evidenced by slowing of weight loss and report of discouragement about lack of rapid progress toward weight goal.

Goals
- Achievement of realistic expectations about amount and pattern of weight loss
- Understanding that total weight is indicative of hydration status as well as fat loss
- Use of nonscale measures of success—eg, changes in how clothes fit as an indication of fat loss

Nutrition Prescription: Continue energy, vitamin, mineral, protein, and physical activity recommendations (registered dietitian would state specific amounts).

Interventions
- Nutrition education, including a review of patterns of post-WLS weight loss and reasonable expectations for weight loss amounts
- Nutrition counseling: self-monitoring—client to graph weight changes over time

Outcome Indicators
- Areas and Level of knowledge (FH-3.1.1)—increased understanding of expected patterns and amounts of weight and fat loss
- Self-monitoring (FH-4.1.4)—weight trends and size changes

Box 5.13 Nutrition Care Process Case Study: A Client with Frequent Diarrhea

Client comes to follow-up appointment and complains of frequent diarrhea associated with intake of sweets and consumption of beverages with meals.

Nutrition Diagnosis: Altered GI function related to malabsorption and nonadherence to post–weight-loss surgery (WLS) guidelines, as evidenced by diarrhea.

Goal: Reduction in or elimination of episodes of diarrhea.[a]

Nutrition Prescription: Registered dietitian recommends specific amount of high-fiber foods and number of servings of complex carbohydrates.

Intervention:
- Food and nutrition delivery: modify distribution and type of food within meals and snacks (ND-1.2):
  ○ Consume small, frequent meals with protein at each meal
  ○ Practice slow, mindful eating and drinking
  ○ Avoid ingestion of liquids within 30 minutes of a solid-food meal
- Food and nutrition delivery: specific food/beverages or groups (ND-1.3):
  ○ Avoid simple sugars
  ○ Increase high-fiber foods and complex carbohydrates

Outcome Indicators
- Types of food/meals (FH-1.3.2.2)—selection per recommendations
- Oral fluid amounts (FH-1.3.1.1)—amount and timing per recommendations
- Self-reported adherence (FH-4.1.1)—reports of food selection indicate adherence to recommendations
- Nutrition-focused physical findings: digestive system (PD-1.1.5)—reduction or elimination of reports of diarrhea

[a]Refer to Appendix G for information about WLS complications and LAGB and suggested treatments.

REFERENCES

1. Pories WJ, Swanson MS, MacDonald KG, et al. Who would have thought it? An operation proves to be the most effective therapy for adult-onset diabetes mellitus. *Ann Surg.* 1995;222:339–352.

2. Buchwald H, Avidor Y, Braunwald E, Jensen MD, Pories W, Fahrbach K, Schoelles K. Bariatric surgery: a systematic review and meta-analysis. *JAMA.* 2004;292:1724–1737.

3. Sugerman HJ, Kellum JM, Engle KM, Wolfe L, Starkey JV, Birkenhauer R, Fletcher P, Sawyer MJ. Gastric bypass for treating severe obesity. *Am J Clin Nutr.* 1992;55(2 Suppl):560S-566S.

4. Rasheid S, Banasiak M, Gallagher SF, Lipska A, Kaba S, Ventimiglia D, Anderson WM, Murr MM. Gastric bypass is an effective treatment for obstructive sleep apnea in patients with clinically significant obesity. *Obes Surg.* 2003;13:58–61.

5. Fritscher LG, Mottin CC, Canani S, Chatkin JM. Obesity and obstructive sleep apnea-hypopnea syndrome: the impact of bariatric surgery. *Obes Surg.* 2007;17:95–99.

6. Brolin RE, Bradley LJ, Wilson AC, Cody RP. Lipid risk profile and weight stability after gastric restrictive operations for morbid obesity. *J Gastroenterol Surg.* 2000;4:464–469.

7. Cummings DE, Weigle DS, Frayo RS, Breen PA, Ma MK, Dellinger EP, Purnell JQ. Plasma ghrelin levels after diet-induced weight loss or gastric bypass surgery. *N Engl J Med.* 2002;346:1623–1630.

8. Mariani LM, Fusco A, Turriziani M, Veneziani A, Marini MA, de Lorenzo A, Bertoli A. Transient increase of plasma ghrelin after laparoscopic adjustable gastric banding in morbid obesity. *Horm Metab Res.* 2005;37:242–245.

9. American Dietetic Association. *International Dietetics & Nutrition Terminology (IDNT) Reference Manual: Standardized Language for the Nutrition Care Process.* 2nd ed. Chicago, IL: American Dietetic Association; 2009.

chapter 6

Long-Term Nutrition Care

This chapter covers nutrition care for the long-term following weight-loss surgery (WLS) (ie, more than 2 years post-WLS).

DESCRIPTION OF CLIENTS

The clients described in this chapter had WLS at least 2 years before the current nutrition care encounter. Nutrition follow-up may or may not have been provided since WLS.

KEY NUTRITION ISSUES

Weight Maintenance and Weight Loss

In this period, clients need to not regain weight lost after WLS. Some clients will also need to lose more weight.

Roux-en-Y Gastric Bypass Clients

Roux-en-Y gastric bypass (RYGBP) clients typically reach their maximum weight loss at approximately 12 to 18 months after WLS, and then regain some weight over the next 3 to 5 years (1–3). Reasons for inadequate weight loss and weight regain after RYGBP have not been well studied. In the absence of anatomical complications, weight regain may be related to decreased frequency of dumping symptoms, resolution of food intolerances, or a return to maladaptive eating behaviors that contributed to the development of obesity (4–6).

Laparoscopic Adjustable Gastric Banding Clients

Compared with RYGBP clients, individuals who had with laparoscopic adjustable gastric banding (LAGB) tend to lose weight more gradually, and weight loss may continue for several years after WLS (7). Failure to achieve optimal weight loss after a LAGB placement has been associated with consumption of calorie-dense liquids that can pass through the stoma without producing satiety (8). LAGB clients may also have a higher tolerance for high-fat and high-calorie foods than clients with RYGBP.

Weight-Loss Expectations

Less than 5% of clients lose 100% of their excess body weight (9). Unrealistic expectations of weight loss are common in clients seeking WLS and can negatively affect long-term adherence to nutrition and health goals (8). In one study, participants reported being disappointed with weight-loss outcomes that providers considered to be successful (9).

Pre-WLS education about expected weight loss is important. However, long-term education, support, and monitoring are also crucial at other times, such as when clients are experiencing the following:

- Cessation of weight loss
- Disappointment with amount of weight lost or post-WLS weight
- Weight regain

Clients should be encouraged to define success from WLS by focusing on factors other than weight loss, such as improvement in or resolution of comorbid conditions, positive psychological changes, and improved quality of life.

Lifestyle and Behavior Changes

To promote further weight loss, weight-loss maintenance, and relapse prevention, clients should be educated about the following:

- Self management
- Use of nonfood strategies to cope with emotions and stress
- Physical activity

Prevention of Vitamin and Mineral Deficits and Deficiencies

Even when educated about potential nutrient deficits and the use of nutrition supplements, many clients do not adhere to the required daily supplementation schedule for micronutrients (9). However, it is important that clients continue to adhere to recommendations for vitamin and mineral supplementation. Deficiencies of iron, vitamin B-12, folate, calcium, and vitamin D can occur after RYGBP and, less commonly, after LAGB. (See Appendix G.)

Disordered Eating Patterns

The registered dietitian (RD) should assess clients to identify any disordered eating patterns that may be affecting the client's ability to maintain weight loss after surgery.

Band Adjustments (LAGB Clients)

The RD should determine whether LAGB clients have had periodic band adjustments when necessary.

Comorbid Conditions

Clients with a history of comorbid conditions of obesity, including diabetes, hypertension, and dyslipidemia, may require continued nutrition management as part of their long-term nutrition care.

NUTRITION ASSESSMENT

At each post-WLS appointment, the RD collects and evaluates a similar set of data. Refer to the assessment section of Chapters 3 and 4 for data to collect and to Appendix F for suggested questions to include in an assessment form. Additional considerations include the following:

- Anthropometric measures: Height should be measured every 5 years.
- Energy requirements: To verify the accuracy of the nutrition prescription for energy, the client's Total Energy Expenditure (TEE) should be reassessed after significant changes in weight and when weight loss does not occur as expected.

NUTRITION DIAGNOSIS

Many nutrition diagnoses and PES statements for the long-term post-WLS period are the same as those described in Chapters 3, 4, and 5. These diagnoses include the following (10):

- Excessive energy intake
- Excessive oral food/beverage intake
- Inadequate vitamin intake
- Inadequate mineral intake
- Self-monitoring deficit
- Limited adherence to nutrition-related recommendations
- Undesirable food choices

- Food and nutrition-related knowledge deficit
- Disordered eating pattern
- Physical inactivity

Refer to earlier chapters for the etiologies and signs and symptoms to use when writing problem, etiology, signs/symptoms (PES) statements for these diagnoses. Boxes 6.1 and 6.2 list additional nutrition diagnoses seen in this time period (10). Box 6.3 offers examples of PES statements for the clients who had WLS more than 2 years ago.

Box 6.1   Nutrition Diagnosis: Involuntary Weight Gain (NC-3.4)

Sample Etiologies
- Undesirable food choices
- Cessation of self-monitoring
- Decreased motivation
- Reduction in social or family support
- Reduced physical activity
- Change in physical health resulting in reduced capacity for physical activity

Common Signs and Symptoms
- Increased weight
- Noticeable change in body fat distribution
- Fat accumulation, excessive subcutaneous fat stores
- Report of changes in recent food intake
- Report of physical inactivity
- Report of use of alcohol

Box 6.2   Nutrition Diagnosis: Inability or Lack of Desire to Manage Self-Care (NI-2.3)

Sample Etiologies
- Lack of support or motivation for long-term changes in behavior
- Underlying issues leading to excess eating, lack of physical activity, and/or lack of self-care

Common Signs and Symptoms
- Inability to interpret data or self-management tools
- Uncertainty regarding changes to be made in response to data in self-monitoring records
- Embarrassment or anger regarding need for self-monitoring

Box 6.3   Sample Diagnosis (PES) Statements

Diagnosis: Inadequate Vitamin B-12 Intake (NI-5.9.1)
Inadequate Vitamin B-12 intake related to lack of compliance with recommendations for taking daily multivitamin supplement and intolerance of red meat, as evidenced by reports of excessive tiredness and fatigue and laboratory signs of megaloblastic anemia.

Diagnosis: Inadequate Calcium Intake (NI-5.10.1)
Inadequate calcium intake related to not taking calcium citrate form of supplement and eating foods low in calcium, as evidenced by high PTH level, low vitamin D level, report of taking carbonate form of calcium supplement, and omission of milk and dairy foods from diet due to lactose intolerance.

Diagnosis: Physical Inactivity (NB-2.1)
Physical inactivity related to increased stress, lack of time, and sedentary job, as evidenced by weight regain and report of increased job demands, working long hours, and lack of physical activity.

Diagnosis: Undesirable Food Choices (NB-1.7)
Undesirable food choices related to consumption of large amounts of soft, high-calorie foods, as evidenced by weight regain and report of daily intake of ice cream, mashed potatoes, and cream soups.

NUTRITION INTERVENTION

The interventions and outcome indicators for the nutrition diagnoses listed earlier in this chapter are similar to those for other WLS time periods and are listed in Chapters 3, 4, and 5 of this pocket guide. Boxes 6.4 and 6.5 list interventions and outcome indicators for the two additional nutrition diagnoses listed in Boxes 6.1 and 6.2, respectively (10).

Box 6.4   Interventions and Outcome Indicators for Involuntary Weight Gain (NC-3.4)

Possible Interventions
- Modify distribution, type, or amount of food and nutrients (ND-1.2):
  - Low-calorie or very-low-calorie diet
  - Reduced fat intake
  - Reduced carbohydrate intake
  - 4–5 meals per day, including breakfast
  - Portion control
  - Meal replacements
- Increased physical activity
- Initial/brief nutrition education:
  - Purpose of nutrition education (E-1.1)
  - Priority modification (E-1.2)
- Comprehensive nutrition education:
  - Purpose of nutrition education (E-2.1)
  - Recommended modification (E-2.2)
  - Advanced or related topics (E-2.3)
  - Result interpretation (E-2.4)
  - Skill development (E-2.5)
- Nutrition counseling: theoretical basis/approach (select) (C-1.1)
- Nutrition counseling: strategies:
  - Motivational interviewing (C-2.1)
  - Goal setting (C-2.2)
  - Self-monitoring (C-2.3)
  - Problem solving (C-2.4)

(continues next page)

**Box 6.4   Interventions and Outcome Indicators for Involuntary
Weight Gain (NC-3.4)** *continued*

Outcome Indicators
- Total energy intake (FH-1.2.1.1)—decreased by 500 kcal/d
  for each pound of desired weight loss per week
- Amount of food (FH-1.3.2.1)—number of food group
  servings per recommendations; reduced portion sizes
- Total fat intake (FH-1.6.1.1)—reduced
- Total carbohydrate (FH-1.6.3.1)—reduced
- Self-reported adherence (FH-4.1.1)—good
- Physical activity:
  - Consistency (FH-6.3.2)—increased
  - Frequency (FH-6.3.3)—increased
  - Duration (FH-6.3.4)—increased
  - Intensity (FH-6.3.6)—increased
  - Strength (FH-6.3.8)—increased
- Body mass index (AD-1.1.5)—reduced
- Weight (AD-1.1.2)—desired amount of weight loss
- Weight change (AD-1.1.4)—weight loss

Box 6.5   Interventions and Outcome Indicators for Inability or Lack of Desire to Manage Self-Care (NB-2.3)

Possible Interventions
- Nutrition counseling: theoretical basis/approach (select) (C-1.1)
- Nutrition counseling: strategies:
  - Motivational interviewing (C-2.1)
  - Goal setting (C-2.2)
  - Problem solving (C-2.4)
  - Social support (C-2.5)
  - Rewards/contingency management (C-2.10)
- Coordination of nutrition care:
  - Team meeting (RC-1.1)
  - Collaboration/referral to other providers (RC-1.3)— consider referral to a mental health professional for assistance in adjusting to short- and long-term psychological changes experienced post-WLS[a]
  - Referral to community agencies/programs (RC-1.4)

Outcome Indicators
- Goal-setting recall (FH-4.1.3)—improved ability; goals set
- Self-monitoring (FH-4.1.4)—improved ability; reported intention to keep records; records kept and brought to appointment
- Self management (FH-4.1.5)—improved
- Ability to build and use social support (FH-4.5.1)— improved; report of support systems established

[a]Data from reference 9 indicate an increased risk of suicide after Roux-en-Y gastric bypass (RYGBP), biliopancreatic diversion (BPD), and biliopancreatic diversion with duodenal switch (DS).

NUTRITION MONITORING AND EVALUATION

After the first year, all WLS clients should be encouraged to have annual visits with the WLS team, including the RD, even in the absence of clinically evident complications and/or intestinal adaptation (11). Additional visits should be scheduled when clients experience life changes, such as a change in employment or in their support system. Frequent appointments may help promote weight-loss maintenance or additional weight loss. In addition, team consultation is needed for special circumstances, including major surgery, severe illnesses, pregnancy, or remote travel (12,13).

REFERENCES

1. Sjöström L, Lindroos AK, Peltonen M, Torgerson J, Bouchard C, Carlsson B, Dahlgren S, Larsson B, Narbro K, Sjöström CD, Sullivan M, Wedel H; Swedish Obese Subjects Study Scientific Group. Lifestyle, diabetes, and cardiovascular risk factors 10 years after bariatric surgery. *N Engl J Med.* 2004;351:2683–2693.

2. Sjöström L, Narbro K, Sjöström CD, Karason K, Larsson B, Wedel H, Lystig T, Sullivan M, Bouchard C, Carlsson B, Bengtsson C, Dahlgren S, Gummesson A, Jacobson P, Karlsson J, Lindroos AK, Lönroth H, Näslund I, Olbers T, Stenlöf K, Torgerson J, Agren G, Carlsson LM; Swedish Obese Subjects Study. Effects of bariatric surgery on mortality in Swedish obese subjects. *N Engl J Med.* 2007;357:741–752.

3. Maclean LD, Rhode BM, Nohr CW. Late outcome of gastric bypass. *Ann Surg.* 2000;231:524–528.

4. Byrne TK. Complications of surgery for obesity. *Surg Clin N Am.* 2001;81:1181–1193.

5. Collene A, Hertzler S. Metabolic outcomes of gastric bypass. *Nutr Clin Pract.* 2003;18:136–140.

6. Adams TD, Gress RE, Smith SC, Halverson RC, Simper SC, Rosamond WD, Lamonte MJ, Stroup AM, Hunt SC. Long-term mortality after gastric bypass surgery. *N Engl J Med.* 2007;357:753–761.

7. O'Brien PE, Dixon JB, Laurie C, Skinner S, Proietto J, McNeil J, Strauss B, Marks S, Schachter L, Chapman L, Anderson M. Treatment of mild to moderate obesity with laparoscopic adjustable gastric banding or an intensive medical program: a randomized trial. *Ann Intern Med.* 2006;144:625–633.

8. Hudson SM, Dixon JB, O'Brien PE. Sweet eating is not a predictor of outcome after Lap-Band placement. Can we finally bury the myth? *Obes Surg.* 2002;12:789–794.

9. Mechanick JI, Kushner RF, Sugerman HJ, for the writing group. Executive summary of the recommendations of the American Association of Clinical Endocrinologists, The Obesity Society, and American Society for Metabolic & Bariatric Surgery medical guidelines for clinical practice for the perioperative nutritional, metabolic, and nonsurgical support of the bariatric surgery patient. *Endocr Pract.* 2008;14:318–336.

10. American Dietetic Association. *International Dietetics & Nutrition Terminology (IDNT) Reference Manual.* 2nd ed. Chicago, IL: American Dietetic Association; 2009.

11. Brolin RE. Gastric bypass. *Surg Clin North Am.* 2001;81:1077–1095.

12. Dixon JB, Dixon ME, O'Brien PE. Birth outcomes in obese women after laparoscopic adjustable gastric banding. *Obstet Gynecol.* 2005;106:965–972.

13. Favretti F, O'Brien PE, Dixon JB. Patient management after LAP-Band placement. *Am J Surg.* 2002;184(suppl):S38–S41.

FURTHER READING

Angrisani L, Lorenzo M, Borrelli V. Laparoscopic adjustable gastric banding versus Roux-en-Y gastric bypass: 5-year results of a prospective randomized trial. *Surg Obes Relat Dis.* 2007;3:127–134.

Bajardi G, Ricevuto G, Mastrandrea G, Branca M, Rinaudo G, Cali F, Diliberti S, Lo Biundo N, Asti V. Surgical treatment of morbid obesity with biliopancreatic diversion and gastric banding: report on an 8-year experience involving 235 cases. *Ann Chir.* 2000; 125:155–162.

Buchwald H, Avidor Y, Braunwald E, Jensen MD, Pories W, Fahrbach K, Schoelles K. Bariatric surgery: a systematic review and meta-analysis. *JAMA.* 2004;292:1724–1737.

Chapman AE, Kiroff G, Game P, Foster B, O'Brien P, Ham J, Maddern GJ. Laparoscopic adjustable gastric banding in the treatment of obesity—a systematic literature review. *Surgery.* 2004;135:326–351.

Jan JC, Hong D, Bardaro SJ, July LV, Patterson EJ. Comparative study between laparoscopic adjustable gastric banding and laparoscopic gastric bypass: single-institution, 5-year experience in bariatric surgery. *Surg Obes Relat Dis*. 2007;3:42–50.

Nguyen NT, Goldman C, Rosenquist CJ, Arango A, Cole CJ, Lee SJ, Wolfe BM. Laparoscopic versus open gastric bypass: a randomized study of outcomes, quality of life, and costs. *Am Surg*. 2001;234:279–291.

O'Brien PE, McPhail T, Chaston TB, Dixon JB. Systematic review of medium-term weight loss after bariatric operations. *Obes Surg*. 2006;16:1032–1040.

Puzziferri N, Austrheim-Smith IT, Wolfe BM, Wilson SE, Nguyen NT. Three-year follow-up of a prospective randomized trial comparing laparoscopic versus open gastric bypass. *Ann Surg*. 2006;243:181–188.

Schauer PR, Ikramuddin S. Laparoscopic surgery for morbid obesity. *Surg Clin North Am*. 2001;81:1145–1179.

Wittgrove AC, Clark GW. Laparoscopic gastric bypass, Roux-en-Y—500 patients: technique and results, with 3–60 month follow-up. *Obes Surg*. 2000;10:233–239.

chapter 7

Adolescent Clients and Weight-Loss Surgery

> **Note:** In 2002, Cincinnati Children's Hospital Medical Center became the first pediatric institution to offer gastric bypass surgery to older adolescents with severe obesity. This multidisciplinary program was designed both to meet the surgical, medical, and nutritional needs of this population, and to address the psychosocial, cognitive, and developmental issues that can affect the success of weight-loss surgery (WLS) in this population (1). Recommendations in this chapter for treating adolescent candidates for WLS are based on practices at this institution and the limited evidence available. As research in this field advances, recommendations may change.

Over the last 30 years, the prevalence of obesity, defined as body mass index (BMI) greater than the 95th percentile for age and sex, has more than doubled for children (ages 6 to 11 years) and tripled for adolescents (ages 12 to 19) (2). Even more concerning is the increase in the *severity* of overweight for children and adolescents (3). This increase has been associated with an increase in obesity-related medical complications, such as type 2 diabetes, obstructive sleep apnea, hypertension, hyperlipidemia, and degenerative joint disease (4), which in the past were health issues largely encountered during adulthood. Therefore, there is an urgent need to seek more aggressive, but safe and effective interventions for youth with severe obesity (BMI ≥ 40).

INITIAL ASSESSMENT

Selection Criteria for Weight-Loss Surgery

An expert panel of surgeons and pediatricians specializing in the treatment of childhood and adolescent obesity developed conservative selection criteria to limit the use of WLS to severely obese adolescents with serious comorbid conditions and to reduce the risk of adverse medical and psychosocial outcomes (Box 7.1) (5). These factors should be taken into consideration as part of an extensive comprehensive assessment by a multidisciplinary team comprised of the surgeon, physicians, a psychologist, a registered dietitian (RD), a social worker, a clinical nurse practitioner, and an exercise physiologist.

Box 7.1 Criteria for Adolescents Being Considered for Gastric Bypass Surgery

- Have failed ≥ 6 months of organized attempts at weight management as determined by their primary care provider
- Have attained or nearly attained physiologic maturity
- Very severely obese (BMI ≥ 40) with serious obesity-related comorbidities or have a BMI ≥ 50 with less severe comorbidities
- Demonstrate commitment to comprehensive medical and psychological evaluations both before and after surgery
- Agree to avoid pregnancy for at least 1 year postoperatively
- Be capable of and willing to adhere to nutritional guidelines postoperatively
- Provide informed assent to surgical treatment
- Demonstrate decisional capacity
- Have a supportive family environment

Source: Reprinted from Inge TH, Krebs NF, Garcia VF, Skelton JA, Guice KS, Strauss RS, Albanese CT, Brandt ML, Hammer LD, Harmon CM, Kane TD, Klish WJ, Rudolph CD, Helmrath MA, Donovan E, Daniels SR. Bariatric surgery for severely overweight adolescents: concerns and recommendations. *Pediatrics*. 2004;14:217–223. Reproduced by permission of the American Academy of Pediatrics.

Role of the Registered Dietitian

During the initial assessment, the RD performs the following tasks:

- Collects baseline anthropometric measurements
- Assesses which weight management strategies were attempted in the past, how long they were used, and, when applicable, why they were discontinued
- Reviews findings with the other members of the multidisciplinary team to determine whether adequate attempts at weight management have been made, and

whether there are any concerns that the client may not comply with the post-WLS dietary regimen

PREOPERATIVE EDUCATION

After the decision is made for the adolescent to proceed with gastric bypass surgery, preoperative education sessions should be offered by individual members of the clinical team, including the RD. A preoperative nutrition education session that is tailored to the needs of adolescents is essential for the following reasons:

- The nutrition education session provides an overview of the progression of the diet stages for the initial 3 months after surgery.
- The session allows the adolescent to learn about the high-protein foods that are acceptable during the first couple of weeks after surgery.
- The session is also an opportunity for the adolescent to taste-test a variety of high-protein drinks (both commercially available products and those prepared with milk, sugar-free instant breakfast, and protein powder) and choose products and flavors they prefer.
- Nutrition education increases the likelihood that the adolescent will comply with the dietary regimen during the initial 3 months after WLS.

ROUX-EN-Y GASTRIC BYPASS PROCEDURE

The Roux-en-Y gastric bypass procedure (RYGBP) is the WLS used in adolescents. Advantages of the RYGBP include the following:

- Advancements in the safety and long-term efficacy have been made in the use of this surgical procedure in morbidly obese adults (mean 61% loss of excess body weight; operative mortality = 0.5%) (6).
- RYGBP may lead to the resolution of or improvement in many obesity-related comorbidities (7).
- Long-term outcomes data in adolescents are comparable to those reported in adults (8,9).

CONCERNS REGARDING WEIGHT-LOSS SURGERY IN ADOLESCENTS

To achieve positive long-term outcomes from WLS, adolescents must adhere to a strict regimen that includes the following (8,9):

- A highly-structured dietary protocol
- Taking daily vitamin and mineral supplements for the rest of their lives
- Sustaining a healthful portion-controlled eating plan and a physically active lifestyle

Adolescents who continually snack on high-fat foods are at risk of regaining most or all of weight lost following WLS. Long-term follow-up care provided by a multidisciplinary team with clinical expertise in working with adolescents is essential and promotes the use of developmentally appropriate behavioral interventions that optimize adherence to the postoperative regimen (1).

NUTRITION PRINCIPLES

Much of what is known about the dietary modifications recommended for adolescents after WLS has been gleaned from the practices of larger, well-established adult surgical programs. Generally, adolescents can follow the same recommendations as adults and benefit from clearly stated guidelines and timeframes for the type, amount, consistency, and texture of food eaten.

Principles for the First Weeks After Surgery

For at least the first 12 weeks after surgery, the adolescent should avoid foods and beverages that contain sugar and those high in fat—these can cause "dumping" symptoms, such as cramps, sweating, heart racing, vomiting, and/or diarrhea. During this period, the client should also avoid carbonated beverages, drinks with caffeine, and alcohol.

Principles for Postsurgery

Protein Intake

After WLS, following a high-protein diet helps maintain lean body mass, promote healing, and minimize hair loss. The client should eat 15 to 20 g of protein from high-quality protein foods at each meal.

When the client begins eating starches, fruits, and vegetables after WLS, the portions of these foods should be limited to very small amounts. (See Table 7.1, later in this chapter.) This will help ensure that protein intake remains adequate. Clients should be encouraged to record the type, amount, and timing for food intake so their protein intake can be assessed.

Other Principles

The client's eating regimen must be strictly controlled after WLS. The health care team should emphasize that the dietary modifications are permanent. Principles to observe include the following:

- Limit the volume of food consumed at each sitting (after 4 weeks have passed since surgery, clients may have up to 1 cup of food per meal).
- Complete each meal in 15 to 20 minutes.
- Stop eating at the first sign of fullness.
- Sip fluids continually between meals. However, do not drink liquids in the 30 minutes before or after a meal.
- Try new foods one at a time, every 2 to 3 days as tolerated. The amount tried should be limited as needed, in order to not exceed the total volume recommended for each stage.

Dietary Progression

Adolescents who have had WLS may take longer to progress from one diet stage to the next. As a result, it is helpful to extend the timeframes of the diet stages, compared with those used with adults who have had WLS, and break them into substages that have specific guidelines. After WLS, adolescents typically receive inpatient treatment for 3 to 5 days. A barium study may be conducted on the first day after WLS to confirm that a leak or pouch obstruction did not occur. If there are no contraindications to feeding, oral fluids (diet stage I) are started.

The stages listed in Table 7.1 are a variation of those recommended for adults (see Appendix B) and are in use at Cincinnati Children's Hospital Medical Center. Sample meal plans for a high-protein diet at two different stages are shown in Tables 7.2 and 7.3 with the corresponding recipes in Table 7.4 and 7.5 (10).

Table 7.1   Recommended Diet Stages for Adolescents After Weight-Loss Surgery

Stage	Description	Duration/Timing
1	**Water and ice chips** • Fluid goal: 1 oz water per hour	• Duration: 1–2 days • Used during hospital stay
2	**Sugar-free clear liquids** • Acceptable fluids: water, broth, sugar-free fruit-flavored drinks, sugar-free ice pops, sugar-free gelatin • Fluid goal: 4–6 oz water/hr; Total: 48–64 oz/d	• Duration: 3–7 days
3	**High-protein liquids/foods with a smooth consistency** • New foods introduced: high-protein drinks (made with nonfat milk or low-fat soy or lactose-free milk), sugar-free pudding, light yogurt (plain or vanilla), low-fat cottage cheese, low-fat ricotta cheese • Protein goal: 50–60 g/d • Fluid goal: 90 oz/d • Calories: 500–600 kcal/d	• Duration: 1–2 weeks • Generally starts after discharge from hospital
4	**Mechanical soft/semi-solid high-protein foods** • New foods introduced: scrambled eggs; minced or ground chicken, turkey, fish, or tofu; tuna; low-fat cheese (not melted) • Food consistency: pureed or chopped into pieces no larger than a pea • Protein goal: ≥ 60 g/d; ≥ 15 g/meal • Volume for solid foods: ½ cup/meal • Meal pattern: 3–4 meals/d • Try new foods one at a time (¼ cup) every 2–3 days	• Duration: 2–3 weeks • Starts ~10–14 days after surgery

(continues next page)

Table 7.1   Recommended Diet Stages for Adolescents After Weight-Loss Surgery (continued)

Stage	Description	Duration/Timing
5	**Soft foods—other protein foods, fruit, vegetables, and grains** • New foods introduced: ◦ Protein foods: shaved deli meats, low-fat melted cheese, lean pork, Canadian bacon, cooked beans ◦ Fruit: soft or canned in own juice; no skin ◦ Vegetables: soft-cooked or canned ◦ Grains: toast, low-sugar cereal, crackers, oatmeal, rice, pasta, mashed potatoes (choose mainly whole grains) • Consistency: Take small bites and chew food well • Protein goal: ≥ 60 g/d • Volume for solid foods: ½–1 cup/meal • Fluid goal: 90 oz/d (emphasis on water) • Meal pattern: 3–4 meals/d	• Duration: 4 weeks • Starts ~4 wk after surgery
6	**Increased texture** • New foods introduced: bread (not toasted); raw fruits and vegetables, including lettuce; nuts, seeds, and popcorn • Protein goal: ≥ 60 g/d • Fluid goal: 64–90 oz/d (emphasis on water) • Volume for solid foods: up to 1 cup/meal • Meal pattern: 3–4 meals/d	• Duration: 4 weeks • Starts ~8 weeks after surgery
7	**All textures and acidities and other high-calorie foods** • Portion-controlled eating plan • New foods introduced: lean red meat, lean pork 100% fruit juice, citrus fruit, olives, avocado, peanut butter, sweets (in moderation), sugar-free carbonated drinks, caffeinated drinks (in moderation) • Protein: ≥ 60 g/d • Volume for solid foods: 1–1½ cups/meal • Meal pattern: 3–4 meals/d	• Duration: lifelong • Starts ~12 weeks after surgery

Protocol is adapted with permission from Cincinnati Children's Hospital Medical Center.

**Table 7.2   Sample Meal Pattern for Stage 3
After Weight-Loss Surgery**

Meal Time	Amount/Food Type	Energy, kcal	Protein, g
8:00 AM	6 oz protein drink	150	15
Noon	½ cup protein-supplemented sugar-free instant pudding	127	12
5:00 PM	6 oz protein drink	150	15
9:00 PM	6 oz protein-supplemented low-fat yogurt (vanilla-flavored or plain)	106	12
	Total	**533 kcal**	**54 g**

Adapted with permission from Kirk S, Inge TH, Daniels SR. Gastric bypass surgery for severely obese adolescents: nutritional considerations. *Pediatric Nutrition: A Building Block for Life* (publication of the Pediatric Nutrition Practice Group). 2005;28(4):1–12.

Table 7.3   Sample Meal Pattern for Stage 5
After Weight-Loss Surgery

Meal Time	Amount/Food Type	Energy, kcal	Protein, g
8:00 AM	2 scrambled eggs (made with 2 Tbsp nonfat milk)	161	15
	¼ slice whole wheat toast (plain)	20	0
Noon	Tuna salad (3 oz water-packed tuna, drained, with 2 Tbsp fat-free mayonnaise)	117	21
	2 whole wheat saltine crackers	26	0
5:00 PM	3 oz minced chicken (with added broth to moisten)	105	21
	2 Tbsp green beans, canned, chopped	6	0
	¼ cup mashed potato	40	1
9:00 PM	½ cup cottage cheese, low-fat, small curd	70	14
	2 Tbsp peaches, canned, drained and chopped	15	0
	Total	**588 kcal**	**72 g**

Adapted with permission from Kirk S, Inge TH, Daniels SR. Gastric bypass surgery for severely obese adolescents: nutritional considerations. *Pediatric Nutrition: A Building Block for Life* (publication of the Pediatric Nutrition Practice Group). 2005;28(4):1–12.

Table 7.4   Recipes for Meal Plans for Stage 3 After Weight-Loss Surgery

Food	Recipe
Protein drink	1 packet sugar-free instant breakfast powder
	⅔ cup nonfat milk
	4 tsp protein powder supplement[a]
Pudding	½ cup sugar-free instant pudding
	1 Tbsp protein powder supplement[a]
Yogurt	6 oz vanilla-flavored or plain low-fat yogurt
	1 Tbsp protein powder supplement[a]

[a]Protein supplement: calcium caseinate or whey protein isolate providing 4 g
protein per Tbsp.
Adapted with permission from Kirk S, Inge TH, Daniels SR. Gastric bypass
surgery for severely obese adolescents: nutritional considerations. *Pediatric
Nutrition: A Building Block for Life* (publication of the Pediatric Nutrition Practice
Group). 2005;28(4):1–12.

Table 7.5   Recipes for Meal Plans for Stage 5 After Weight-Loss Surgery

Food	Recipe
Scrambled eggs	2 eggs
	¼ cup skim milk
	1½ Tbsp protein powder supplement[a]
Tuna salad	3 oz can tuna packed in water
	2 Tbsp + 2 tsp fat-free mayonnaise
	1 Tbsp protein powder supplement[a]
Minced chicken in broth	½ cup minced chicken (skinless, boneless, boiled, white meat only)
	3 Tbsp chicken broth
Mashed potatoes	¼ cup mashed boiled potato with nonfat milk (no added fat)
	2 tsp protein powder supplement[a]
Cottage cheese	½ cup cottage cheese (small curd)
	1 Tbsp protein powder supplement[a]

[a]Protein supplement: calcium caseinate or whey protein isolate providing 4 g
protein per Tbsp.
Adapted with permission from Kirk S, Inge TH, Daniels SR. Gastric bypass
surgery for severely obese adolescents: nutritional considerations. *Pediatric
Nutrition: A Building Block for Life* (publication of the Pediatric Nutrition Practice
Group). 2005;28(4):1–12.

Vitamin and Mineral Supplementation

After WLS, lifelong daily vitamin and mineral supplementation is recommended. Supplements should include the following:

- A sugar-free multivitamin and mineral supplement (for menstruating females, use a prenatal supplement with iron)
- Vitamin B-12: 500 mcg sublingual or 1,000 mcg by injection every 4 to 6 weeks
- Calcium: 1,500 mg/d is recommended; choose a calcium citrate form for optimal absorption
- Vitamin B-1 (thiamin): 50 mg/d for the first 6 months after surgery

Cases of beriberi resulting from vitamin B-1 deficiency have been reported in adolescents who experience post-WLS vomiting. This may suggest that, compared with adults who have had WLS, adolescent WLS clients are at greater risk of beriberi due to thiamin malabsorption. However, it also could be that the adolescents in the case reports did not comply with supplementation recommendations. Strict adherence to dietary and nutrition supplement regimens can prevent such deficiencies (11,12).

MONITORING AND EVALUATION

After WLS, follow-up with a health care team can help the adolescent integrate the restricted dietary plan and continual need to sip fluids throughout the day into his or her daily life. In addition, long-term follow-up helps the team monitor and evaluate whether the following goals are being met:

- Nutrition is sufficient to preserve lean body mass while optimizing loss of body fat.
- The exercise routine includes both aerobic and weight resistance activities.

Inpatient

The role of the RD during the client's hospital stay is outlined in Box 7.2.

Box 7.2   Role of the Registered Dietitian in an Inpatient Setting

- Ensure that the adolescent and family members understand the progression of the diet used during and immediately after the hospital stay.
- Ensure that self-monitoring of fluid intake has begun.
- Provide ample opportunity for questions and answers.
- Confirm that the family has necessary products and equipment to advance dietary stages after discharge.
- Remind clients to expand daily tracking to include vitamin/mineral supplements, food and drink consumed, and physical activity after discharge.

Outpatient

Postsurgical follow-up involves a clinical team of a surgeon, a nurse, an RD, and an exercise specialist. A behavioral psychologist should also meet with clients postoperatively on an as-needed basis. See Box 7.3 for the role of the RD.

Box 7.3   Role of the Registered Dietitian at Follow-up Visits

- Reviews compliance with the following:
  - Assigned diet stage
  - Volume of food and drink consumed
  - Timing of meals
  - Amount of protein and energy intake
  - Daily vitamin and mineral supplements
- Identifies food cravings and any adverse reactions associated with intake of food or drink
- Assesses readiness to advance to the next dietary stage
- Uses behavioral tools, such as goal-setting, contracts, and self-monitoring, to reinforce the anatomic and physiologic effects of the surgery, so that the desired behaviors become more of a habit and not simply a reaction to the altered anatomy

Follow-up Schedule

In the first year after surgery, follow-up visits are scheduled at 2 weeks, 6 weeks, 3 months, 6 months, and 1 year. A 9-month follow-up visit may also be scheduled, depending on the individual client's adjustment to the diet and exercise regimen. In the second year after surgery, two follow-up visits are scheduled (at 18 and 24 months). Annual visits are recommended after year 2.

Data Collected at Follow-Up Visits

In addition to follow-up from their WLS team, clients also meet with their primary care physician at their 6-month, 1-year and 2-year follow-up visits. Laboratory tests and an echocardiogram are obtained at these appointments.

Weight and height measurements are obtained at each visit. Body composition should also be periodically assessed by dual energy x-ray absorptiometry (DEXA). DEXA data are generally obtained at the 6-month, 1-year, and 2-year follow-up visits.

REFERENCES

1. Inge TH, Garcia V, Daniels S, Langford L, Kirk S, Roehrig H, Amin R, Zeller M, Hige K. A multidisciplinary approach to the adolescent bariatric surgical patient. *J Pediatr Surg*. 2004;39: 442–447.

2. Ogden CL, Flegal KM, Carroll MD, Johnson CL. Prevalence and trends in overweight among U.S. children and adolescents, 1999–2000. *JAMA*. 2002;288:1728–1732.

3. Strauss RS, Pollack HA. Epidemic increase in childhood overweight, 1986–1998. *JAMA*. 2001;291:2847–2850.

4. Dietz WH. Health consequences of obesity in youth: childhood predictors of adult disease. *Pediatrics*. 1998;101:518–525.

5. Inge TH, Krebs NF, Garcia VF, Skelton JA, Guice KS, Strauss RS, Albanese CT, Brandt ML, Hammer LD, Harmon CM, Kane TD, Klish WJ, Rudolph CD, Helmrath MA, Donovan E, Daniels SR. Bariatric surgery for severely overweight adolescents: concerns and recommendations. *Pediatrics*. 2004;14:217–223.

6. Horgan S, Holterman MJ, Jacobsen GR, Browne AF, Berger RA, Moser F, Holterman AX. Laparoscopic adjustable gastric banding for the treatment of adolescent morbid obesity in the United States: a safe alternative to gastric bypass. *J Pediatr Surg*. 2005;40:86–90.

7. Buchwald H, Avidor Y, Braunwald E, Jensen MD, Pories W, Fahrbach K, Schoelles K. Bariatric surgery: a systematic review and meta-analysis. *JAMA*. 2004;292:1724–1737.

8. Sugerman HJ, Sugerman EL, DeMaria EJ, Kellum JM, Kennedy C, Mowery Y, Wolfe LG. Bariatric surgery for severely obese adolescents. *J Gastrointestinal Surg*. 2003;7:102–108.

9. Rand CS, MacGregor AM. Adolescents having obesity surgery: a 6-year follow-up. *South Med J*. 1994;87:1208–1213.

10. Kirk S, Inge TH, Daniels SR. Gastric bypass surgery for severely obese adolescents: nutritional considerations. *Pediatric Nutrition: A Building Block for Life* (newsletter). 2005;28(4):1–12.

11. Alvarex-Leite JL. Nutrient deficiencies secondary to bariatric surgery. *Curr Opin Clin Nutr Metab Care*. 2004;7:569–575.

12. Towbin A, Inge TH, Garcia VF, Roehrig HR, Clements RH, Harmon CM, Daniels SR. Beriberi after gastric bypass surgery in adolescence. *Pediatrics*. 2004;145:263–267.

chapter 8

Nutrition Support After Weight-Loss Surgery

Clients who have had weight-loss surgery (WLS) and require nutrition support have nutrition concerns that are in many ways similar to those of other nutrition support patients. While access for feeding tubes may be difficult, energy and protein requirements will depend on the client's medical condition, and pre-existing vitamin and mineral deficiencies.

DESCRIPTION OF CLIENTS

Critically ill patients may be intubated, sedated (possibly with lipid-containing propofol), at risk of aspiration, or hypermetabolic. Nutrition support may be required when clients are unable to consume adequate oral food and/or beverages to meet estimated nutrient requirements. The appropriate type of nutrition support may depend on the setting in which the client receives care (ie, acute, long-term, or home care).

KEY NUTRITION ISSUES

When administering nutrition support to individuals who have had WLS, the clinician must be aware of the potential for the following:

- Impaired ability to absorb nutrients

- Dehydration
- Protein-energy malnutrition

NUTRITION ASSESSMENT

Biochemical Data, Medical Tests, and Procedures

The nutrition assessment should include laboratory data for the following:

- Blood glucose: the client may need an IV insulin glucose tolerance test
- Blood urea nitrogen and creatinine
- Liver function tests (LFTs) and total bilirubin: if results from LFTs are abnormal and the client is more than 6 months post-WLS, check serum levels of fat-soluble vitamins
- Electrolytes, especially in clients who need total parenteral nutrition (TPN)
- Serum vitamin B-12 if client is > 6 months post-WLS
- Serum thiamin

Anthropometric Measurements

Anthropometric assessment should note the client's height, weight, body mass index (BMI).

Nutrition-Focused Physical Findings

Refer to Table 8.1 for the physical examination components of the nutrition assessment.

Table 8.1   Physical Examination Findings Relevant to Nutrition Assessment of Nutrition Support Patients

Category	Assess
Vital signs	• Blood pressure
	• Pulse
	• Respiration
Cardiopulmonary	• Ability to breathe without assistance/mechanical ventilation
	• Pulmonary edema
Gastrointestinal	• Nausea
	• Vomiting
	• Bowel function
	• Low vs high output fistulas
	• Length of functional GI tract (> 100 cm of small bowel)
	• Inputs and outputs (I & Os)
Head and neck	• Mouth and throat: glossitis, bleeding gums, cracked lips
	• Eyes: sunken
	• Tongue
Neurological	• Confusion
	• Coma
Skin and nails	• Skin: dry, decreased elasticity, bruising, flushing, cold at extremities
	• Pressure ulcers and/or wounds
	• Nails: pale nail beds

Food/Nutrition-Related History

The food and nutrition history should include the client's food and nutrient intake, food tolerance, and fluid intake. Assessment should also note the following intake patterns:

- Oral intake < 50% of required nutrient intake for 5 to 7 days
- NPO for 7 to 10 days

- Unable to obtain > 50% of energy needs from enteral nutrition

Client History

Medication and Supplement Use

In the client history portion of the nutrition assessment, evaluate the client's use of prescription and over-the-counter medications. Include medications currently being taken as well as those used before admission. Also note any supplements (protein, vitamins, minerals, fiber, or herbals) used by the client.

Medical History

A medical history evaluating the following should be part of the nutrition assessment:

- Comorbidities
- Surgeries—for WLS, note the date and type of WLS procedure as well as weight change since WLS and the percentage of excess body weight loss
- Other treatments
- Reason for admission
- Current medical condition—eg, severe dysphagia, presence of sepsis, or need for additional surgery

Energy and Protein Needs

To assess the client's energy needs, use indirect calorimetry, if available, to measure resting energy expenditure. An accurate assessment is important to avoid under- or overfeeding.

If indirect calorimetry is not available, estimate energy needs. If predictive equations are needed for mechanically ventilated, critically ill obese patients, consider using the Ireton-Jones 1992 or Penn State 1998 equations because they have the best predictive accuracy of equations studied. For more information on determining energy requirements for critically ill patients, refer to the ADA Evidence Analysis Library's Critical Illness Nutrition Practice Guideline (1).

Estimation of protein needs is difficult in overweight and obese critically ill patients. Studies with obese patients suggest that hypocaloric, high-protein nutrition support (1.5 to 2 g protein per kilogram of ideal body weight) may achieve nitrogen balance in patients without renal or liver disease (2–4). However, larger clinical studies are needed to confirm these results.

Additional Factors Related to Obesity

Nutrition assessment of obese clients who require nutrition support should take into account the following:

- There is a lack of scientific evidence to support use of adjusted body weight to estimate metabolically active tissue in ill obese patients.
- Insulin resistance or diabetes increases risk for hyperglycemia in acutely stressed obese clients (5,6).
- Hyperinsulinemia and hemodynamic factors increase the risk for fluid retention and volume overload in acutely stressed obese clients (5,6).

NUTRITION DIAGNOSIS

Some nutrition diagnoses and problem, etiology, signs/symptoms (PES) statements for post-WLS clients who need nutrition support may be the same as those described in Chapters 4, 5, and 6. These diagnoses include the following:

- Inadequate vitamin intake

- Inadequate mineral intake
- Inadequate protein intake
- Inadequate fluid intake

Boxes 8.1 and 8.2 list additional nutrition diagnoses seen in clients who require nutrition support, with sample etiologies, and likely signs and symptoms (7). Box 8.3 offers examples of PES statements.

Box 8.1   Nutrition Diagnosis: Inadequate Oral Food/Beverage Intake (NI-2.1)

Sample Etiologies
- Increased nutrient needs due to trauma or prolonged catabolic illness
- Food intolerances
- Altered gastrointestinal function due to weight-loss surgery

Signs and Symptoms
- Report or observation of insufficient intake of energy, vitamins, minerals and/or high-quality protein from diet when compared with requirements
- Protein and/or nutrient malabsorption

**Box 8.2   Nutrition Diagnosis: Inadequate Intake from
Enteral/Parenteral Nutrition (NI-2.3)**

Sample Etiologies
- Altered absorption of nutrients, eg, due to surgery
- Altered metabolism of nutrients
- Lack of, compromised, or incorrect access for delivering
  enteral nutrition (EN) or parenteral nutrition (PN)
- Increased demand for nutrients, eg, wound healing, chronic
  infection, multiple fractures (trauma)
- Altered gastrointestinal function
- Intolerance of EN/PN
- Infusion volume not reached or schedule for infusion
  interrupted

Common Signs and Symptoms
- Altered vitamin/mineral laboratory values
- Clinical evidence of vitamin/mineral deficiency
- Unintentional weight loss
- Evidence of dehydration
- Loss of skin integrity, delayed wound healing, or pressure
  ulcers
- Physical signs of malnutrition
- Nausea, vomiting, diarrhea
- Inadequate volume of EN/PN compared with estimated or
  measured (indirect calorimetry) needs
- Feeding tube or venous access in wrong position or removed

Box 8.3   Sample Nutrition Diagnoses (PES Statements)

Nutrition Diagnosis: Inadequate Oral Food/Beverage Intake (NI-2.1)
Inadequate oral food/beverage intake *(problem)* related to injuries sustained in a post-weight-loss surgery motor vehicle accident *(etiology)*, as evidenced by observation of inability to consume oral nutrition while on mechanical ventilation *(signs/symptoms)*

Nutrition Diagnosis: Inadequate Intake from Enteral/Parenteral Nutrition (NI-2.3)
Inadequate intake from enteral/parenteral nutrition *(problem)* related to frequent interruptions of infusion schedule *(etiology)*, as evidenced by delayed wound healing and insufficient infusion of EN compared with requirements *(signs/symptoms)*

NUTRITION INTERVENTION

Goal Setting

In the intervention step of the Nutrition Care Process, the registered dietitian (RD) defines goals to resolve nutrition diagnoses and/or to reduce or eliminate the signs and symptoms of nutrition diagnoses. Examples of these goals include the following:

- Infusion of ordered EN/parenteral nutrition (PN) to meet nutrient needs
- Normalization of or improvement in laboratory values
- Correction of vitamin/mineral deficiencies
- Wound healing

Nutrition Prescription

The RD determines the nutrition prescription for energy, protein, fluid, vitamins, and minerals.

Strategies

Nutrition intervention strategies such as the following are selected to meet the goals and nutrition prescription:

- Assess the need for nutrition support.
- If client is on propofol, count ~1 kcal per mL of fat as an energy source.
- Check serum vitamin B-12 and provide supplementation as needed.
- Provide calcium supplementation, orally or in TPN
- Give iron, folate, and multivitamins as needed.
- Determine appropriateness of EN vs PN to meet nutrient needs. (Refer to Box 8.4 [8] and Table 8.2.)
- For EN patients, recommend enteral tube location (see Box 8.5), select formula type, and define infusion schedule (see reference 9 for more information).
- For PN patients, write PN orders (for more information, see reference 9).
- Identify laboratory values, anthropometric measurements, food and nutrition history, and client data to monitor and evaluate.
- Determine frequency of monitoring and evaluation.

Box 8.4   Indications for Enteral or Parenteral Nutrition

When to Use Enteral Nutrition
- Patient has protein-energy malnutrition with inadequate oral nutrient intake for 5 or more days and intake is not expected to improve.
- Oral intake provides < 50% of required nutrients for 5–7 days.
- Patient has functional gastrointestinal (GI) tract (> 100 cm of small bowel).
- Patient requires prolonged mechanical ventilation.
- Patient has severe dysphagia/swallowing difficulties.
- Patient is in coma.
- Patient has low output enterocutaneous fistulas.
- Patient has any of the following complications:
  - Sepsis with gastric or intestinal access
  - Abscess without affecting motility or GI tract
  - Respiratory failure requiring endotracheal intubation without affecting GI tract
  - Fistula with distal feeding access, low output

When to Use Parenteral Nutrition
- Patient is NPO, inadequate intake is expected for 7–10 days, and patient is unable to be fed enterally.
- Patient is severely malnourished, requires major surgery, and is unable to be fed enterally.
- Patient has severe postoperative complications and is unable to be fed enterally.
- Less than 50% of calorie needs can be given from tube feeding for > 7–10 days.
- Patient has high output fistulas.
- Patient has no GI motility.

Source: Data are from reference 8.

Table 8.2   Advantages and Disadvantages of Enteral and Parenteral Nutrition

	Advantages	*Disadvantages*
Enteral nutrition	• Low metabolic response to stress • Improved glycemic control • Reduced infections • Increased GALT • Cost effective	• GI intolerance • Access, although some patients may tolerate oral gastric and nasogastric tubes • Distention • Diarrhea • Aspiration risk •
Parenteral nutrition	• Able to provide 100% of calorie, protein, vitamin, and mineral needs • Access • Source of nutrition when GI tract in unavailable for enteral feeding • No aspiration risk	• Immunosuppressive • Risk for line infection • If energy intake exceeds energy needs, risk of hyperglycemia or hepatic steatosis • Poor amino acid ratio—no glutamine • Excessive IV n-6 fatty acids, which are proinflammatory • Nonluminal delivery, which compromises mucosal barrier and atrophies GALT • Potential for long-term complications, such as metabolic bone disease

Abbreviations: GI, gastrointestinal; GALT, gut-associated lymphoid tissue; IV, intravenous.

Box 8.5   Selection of Enteral Nutrition Tube Locations in Weight-Loss Patients

- Gastrostomy tube is used if the remnant stomach has adequate motility.
- Jejunostomy is used if reflux or residuals are present with gastrostomy. This is placed past the Y limb in Roux-en-Y gastric bypass patients.
- Small bowel feeding tube is placed past the pouch.

MONITORING AND EVALUATION

Boxes 8.6 and 8.7 list nutrition diagnoses for WLS clients who require nutrition support, with possible nutrition interventions and outcome indicators that can be used to evaluate the effectiveness of the interventions in the monitoring and evaluation step of the Nutrition Care Process (7). Consult references 7 and 9 for additional information on monitoring patients on EN and PN.

Box 8.6   Interventions and Outcome Indicators for Inadequate Oral Food/Beverage Intake (NI-2.1)

Possible Interventions
- Enteral nutrition (EN) or parenteral nutrition (PN):
  - Initiate EN or PN (ND-1.2)
  - Modify rate, concentration, composition, or schedule (ND-2.2)
  - Insert enteral feeding tube (ND-2.4)
- Vitamin and mineral supplements:
  - Vitamins (ND-3.2.3)
  - Minerals (ND-3.2.4)

Outcome Indicators
- Total energy intake (FH-1.2.1.1)
- EN and PN intake (FH-1.4):
  - Access (FH-1.4.1.1)
  - Formula/solution (FH-1.4.1.2)
  - Initiation (FH-1.4.1.4)
  - Rate/schedule (FH-1.4.1.5)
- Total protein intake (FH-1.6.2.1)
- Vitamin intake (FH-1.7.1)
- Mineral intake (FH-1.7.2)

Box 8.7   Interventions and Outcome Indicators for Inadequate Intake from Enteral/Parenteral Nutrition (NI-2.3)

Possible Interventions
- Enteral nutrition (EN) or parenteral nutrition (PN):
  - Initiate EN or PN (ND-2.1)
  - Modify rate, concentration, composition, or schedule (ND-2.2)
- Vitamin and mineral supplements:
  - Vitamins (ND-3.2.3)
  - Minerals (ND-3.2.4)

Outcome Indicators
- Total energy intake (FH-1.2.1.1)
- EN and PN intake (FH-1.4):
  - Access (FH-1.4.1.1)
  - Formula/solution (FH-1.4.1.2)
  - Initiation (FH-1.4.1.4)
  - Rate/schedule (FH-1.4.1.5)
- Total protein intake (FH-1.6.2.1)
- Vitamin intake (FH-1.7.1)
- Mineral intake (FH-1.7.2)

REFERENCES

1. American Dietetic Association Evidence Analysis Library: Critical Illness Evidence-Based Nutrition Practice Guideline. http://www.adaevidencelibrary.com. Accessed May 13, 2008.
2. Dickerson RN, Rosoto EF, Mullen JL. Net protein anabolism with hypocaloric parenteral nutrition in obese stressed patients. *Am J Clin Nutr.* 1986;44:747–755.
3. Burge JC, Goon A, Choban PS, Flancbaum L. Efficacy of hypocaloric TPN in hospitalized obese patients: a prospective, double-blind randomized trial. *JPEN J Parenter Enteral Nutr.* 1994;18:203–207.
4. Choban PS, Burger JC, Scales D, Flancbaum L. Hypo-energetic nutrition support in hospitalized obese patients. A simplified method for clinical application. *Am J Clin Nutr.* 1997;66:546–550.

5. Dickerson RN. Specialized nutrition support in the hospitalized obese patient. *Nutr Clin Pract.* 2004;19:245–254.

6. Choban PS, Dickerson RN. Morbid obesity and nutrition support: is bigger different? *Nutr Clin Pract.* 2005;20:480–487.

7. American Dietetic Association. *International Dietetics & Nutrition Terminology (IDNT) Reference Manual.* 2nd ed. Chicago, IL: American Dietetic Association; 2009.

8. A.S.P.E.N. Board of Directors. Guidelines for the use of parenteral and enteral nutrition in adult and pediatric patients. *JPEN J Parenter Enteral Nutr.* 2002;26(1 Suppl):1SA-138SA.

9. Gottschlich M, ed. *Nutrition Support Core Curriculum: A Case-Based Approach—The Adult Patient.* Silver Spring, MD: American Society for Parenteral and Enteral Nutrition; 2007.

FURTHER READING

Alaverez-Leite JI. Nutrient deficiencies secondary to bypass surgery. *Curr Opin Clin Nutr Metab Care.* 2004;7:569–575.

Alexander JW, Goodman H. Gastric bypass in chronic renal failure and renal transplant. *Nutr Clin Pract.* 2007;22:16–22.

Buchwald H, Avidor Y, Braunwald E, Jensen MD, Pories W, Fahrbach K, Schoelles K. Bariatric surgery: a systematic review and meta-analysis. *JAMA.* 2004;292:1724–1737.

Halaverson JD. Micronutrient deficiencies after gastric bypass for morbid obesity. *Am Surg.* 1986;52:594–598.

Saadeh S. Nonalcoholic fatty liver disease and obesity. *Nutr Clin Pract.* 2007;22:1–10.

Shikora SA, Kim JJ, Tarnoff ME. Nutrition and gastrointestinal complications of bariatric surgery. *Nutr Clin Pract.* 2007;22:29–40.

Torosian MH. Perioperative nutrition support for patients undergoing gastrointestinal surgery: critical analysis and recommendations. *World J Surg,* 1999;23:565–569.

chapter 9

Pregnancy After Weight-Loss Surgery

TIMING OF PREGNANCY AFTER WEIGHT-LOSS SURGERY

Most experts recommend that women avoid pregnancy for 12 to 18 months after any type of weight-loss surgery (WLS). However, women have delivered healthy babies in the first year after WLS (1).

POSSIBLE PREGNANCY COMPLICATIONS RELATED TO WEIGHT-LOSS SURGERY

Case reports of maternal and infant morbidity and mortality have been noted both in early and late pregnancy (2–5). Perhaps the most notable potential serious complication is that of small bowel obstruction or herniation after WLS.

Women who become pregnant after biliopancreatic diversion (BPD) warrant close clinical observation because the rates of low-birth-weight (LBW) and small-for-gestational-age (SGA) infant births associated with BPD are higher than those for other WLS procedures (6).

OBESITY-RELATED RISKS IN PREGNANCY

Many women who become pregnant after WLS remain clinically obese despite substantial weight loss (7). Studies

suggest that obese women who become pregnant after
Roux-en-Y gastric bypass (RYGBP) and laparoscopic
adjustable gastric banding (LAGB) have fewer obesity-
related complications than pregnant obese women in the
general population (8,9). However, the reproductive complications of maternal obesity are well documented.
Women in all three classes of obesity have significantly
higher rates of the following pregnancy complications
compared with normal-weight pregnant women (10):

- Gestational hypertension
- Pre-eclampsia
- Gestational diabetes mellitus
- Preterm delivery
- Macrosomic infants

Despite these risks, pregnancy rates for women in the
United States with class III obesity (body mass index
[BMI] ≥ 40) have increased substantially in recent
decades, from approximately 2% in 1980 to more than
10% in 2000 (11).

MEDICAL NUTRITION THERAPY GOALS

Nutrition goals for women who become pregnant after
WLS include the following:

- Adequate weight gain to promote fetal growth (see
  Table 9.1) (12)
- Vitamin and mineral supplementation to correct or
  prevent deficiencies
- Education on nutrition during pregnancy and lacta-
  tion and post-WLS issues that affect pregnancy

Table 9.1   Weight Gain Recommendations During Pregnancy

Body Mass Index[a]	Recommended Weight Gain, lb
< 19.8	28–40
19.8–26	25–35
> 26–29	15–25
> 29	15

[a]Use the woman's body mass index at the beginning of her pregnancy to determine appropriate weight gain.
Source: Data are from reference 12.

NUTRITION ASSESSMENT

Anthropometric Measurements

The nutrition assessment should include the following anthropometric information about the client:

- Height
- Weight
- Pre-gravid BMI
- Percentage of excess body weight loss
- Amount of weight loss or weight gain during pregnancy

Biochemical Data, Medical Tests, and Procedures

In the nutrition assessment, use normal laboratory values for pregnancy (see Table 9.2 [13]) and evaluate the following data:

- Comprehensive metabolic profile
- Complete blood count
- Results from serum iron panel
- Serum thiamin, vitamins B-6 and B-12, and folate
- Serum levels of fat soluble vitamins (A, D, and K) and zinc, in clients with WLS procedures associated with malabsorption

Table 9.2 Common Laboratory Values During Pregnancy

Laboratory Test	Normal Values for Nonpregnant Women	Normal Values for Pregnant Women
Total protein, g/dL	6.8–8.5	6.8
Albumin, g/dL	3.5–5	2.5–4.5
Prealbumin, mg/dL	17–39	19–29
Retinol-binding protein, mg/dL	2.7–7.6	2.5–4
Blood urea nitrogen, mg/dL	5–24	4–12
Creatinine, mg/dL	0.7–1.3	0.4–0.9
Fasting glucose, mg/dL	65–115	65–100
2-hr postprandial glucose, mg/dL	< 110	< 120
Calcium, mEq/L	9–10.5	8.4–10.4
Phosphorus, mg/dL	2.5–4.5	2.3–4.6
Alkaline phosphatase, U/L	0–95	35–150
Cholesterol, mg/dL	< 200	177–345
Triglycerides, mg/dL	< 250	120–400
Folic acid, ng/mL	5–21	4–14
Iron, mcg/dL	60–160	> 60
Ferritin, mcg/L	10–150	> 20
Total iron-binding capacity (TIBC), mcg/dL	250–460	300–600
TIBC saturation, %	30	> 20
Vitamin B-12, pg/mL	199–732	Decreased (ie, may be below nonpregnant normal value)
Zinc (mcg/dL)	65–115	55–80

Adapted with permission from Blankenship JD, Turnier-Lamoureaux N. Pregnancy 101: laboratory assessment. *The Women's Health and Reproductive Nutrition Report.* 2005:5;6–7.

Pregnant women who had RYGBP should not be given an oral glucose tolerance test (OGTT). The test may cause dumping syndrome, which makes it difficult to interpret the results and creates an undesirable and possibly dangerous situation during pregnancy. Clients with LAGB may be able to tolerate the OGTT without dumping syndrome, but they may not be able to drink the full carbohydrate load needed for the OGTT.

Nutrition-Focused Physical Findings

The RD should assess the client for the following:

- Changes in hair, skin, nails
- Changes in memory (eg, memory lapses)
- Numbness or tingling in hands and/or feet
- Burning sensation in feet
- Other clinical symptoms of nutrition-related problems/conditions

Food/Nutrition-Related History

Assessment of the client's food and nutrient intake should include the following:

- Current intake patterns
- Energy and protein intake
- Compliance with supplementation recommendations
- Disordered eating, including pica, food aversions, binge eating, bulimia, or anorexia

NUTRITION DIAGNOSIS

Potential nutrition diagnoses during pregnancy include the following:

- Inadequate energy intake (which may lead to inadequate weight gain during pregnancy)
- Excessive weight gain—note: the only published report of this occurred in a patient with LAGB who had prophylactic saline removal without any indication for doing so (5)
- Inadequate protein intake

- Inadequate vitamin intake—hyperemesis during pregnancy increases risk for thiamin insufficiency beyond the risk generally associated with gastric bypass and adjustable banding procedures
- Inadequate mineral intake

NUTRITION INTERVENTION

Box 9.1 shows an example of a nutrition prescription for a woman who had WLS and is now pregnant.

Box 9.1   Nutrition Prescription for Pregnant Woman with History of Weight-Loss Surgery

---

- Protein: 1.1 g per kilogram of non-pregnant ideal body weight for height or 71 g/d
- Energy: 300 to 500 kcal more than amount needed for gastric bypass maintenance; usually at least 1,500 to 1,800 kcal/d. Energy should be adequate to promote desired weight gain and optimize fetal growth.[a]
- Fat: Dietary source of DHA is desirable; evaluate cold water fish intake and consider a DHA supplement if consuming less than 2 servings per week. Note: this recommendation meets the Food and Drug Administration safety guideline to limit fish consumption to two 6-oz. servings (12 oz. total) during pregnancy and lactation.
- Vitamin and mineral supplementation to optimize fetal growth.

---

[a]Refer to Table 9.1 for the Institute of Medicine's weight gain recommendations.

Intervention Strategies to Increase Intake

The following practices may help increase intake:

- Eating five or six small meals that include a protein source each day

- Having three daily servings of milk, dairy foods, or a milk alternative such as fortified soy milk
- Avoiding consumption of liquids with meals
- Choosing nutrient-dense foods

Oral protein supplements may be appropriate for some women. Consider nutrition support if poor weight gain or weight loss is noted or there is inadequate fetal growth.

LAGB clients, especially those with prolonged nausea and vomiting, may benefit from saline adjustment.

Nutrition Education

Topics for education include the following:

- Weight gain during pregnancy
- Nutrient requirements of pregnancy, including vitamin and mineral supplementation
- Management of common complications
- Breastfeeding
- Realistic postpartum weight-loss goals

MONITORING AND EVALUATION

The RD should monitor the following in pregnant women with a history of WLS:

- Weight and weight gain
- Intake (monitor through food records)
- Urinary ketones

REFERENCES

1. Dao T, Kuhn J, Ehmer D, Fisher T, McCarty T. Pregnancy outcomes after gastric-bypass surgery. *Am J Surg*. 2006;192:762–766.

2. Kakarla N, Dailey C, Marino T, Shikora SA, Chelmow D. Pregnancy after gastric bypass surgery and internal hernia formation. *Obstet Gynecol*. 2005;105:1195–1198.

3. Charles A, Domingo S, Goldfadden A, Fader J, Lampmann R, Mazzeo R. Small bowel ischemia after Roux-en-Y gastric bypass complicated by pregnancy: a case report. *Am Surg*. 2005;71:231–234.

4. Moore KA, Ouyang DW, Whang EE. Maternal and fetal deaths after gastric bypass surgery for morbid obesity. *N Engl J Med*. 2004;351:721–722.

5. Martin LF, Finigan KM, Nolan TE. Pregnancy after adjustable gastric banding. *Obstet Gynecol*. 2000;95:927–930.

6. Friedman D, Cuneo S, Valenzano M, Marinari GM, Adami GF, Gianetta E, Traverso E, Scopinaro N. Pregnancies in an 18-year follow-up after biliopancreatic diversion. *Obes Surg*. 1995;5:308–313.

7. Sheiner E, Levy A, Silverberg D, Menes TS, Levy I, Katz M, Mazor M. Pregnancy after bariatric surgery is not associated with adverse perinatal outcome. *Am J Obstet Gynecol*. 2004;190:1335–1340.

8. Wittgrove AC, Jester L, Wittgrove P, Clark GW. Pregnancy following gastric bypass for morbid obesity. *Obes Surg*. 1998;8:461–464; discussion, 465–466.

9. Dixon JB, Dixon ME, O'Brien PE. Birth outcomes in obese women after laparoscopic adjustable gastric banding. *Obstet Gynecol*. 2005;106:965–972.

10. Nuthalapaty FS, Rouse DJ. The impact of obesity on obstetrical practice and outcome. *Clin Obstet Gynecol*. 2004;47:898–913.

11. Weiss JL, Malone FD, Emig D, Ball RH, Nyberg DA, Comstock CH, Saade G, Eddleman K, Carter SM, Craigo SD, Carr SR, D'Alton ME; FASTER Research Consortium. Obesity, obstetric complications and cesarean delivery rate—a population-based screening study. *Am J Obstet Gynecol*. 2004;190:1091–1097.

12. Institute of Medicine. *Nutrition During Pregnancy and Lactation*. Washington, DC: National Academy Press; 1992.

13. Blankenship JD, Turnier-Lamoureaux N. Pregnancy 101: laboratory assessment. *The Women's Health and Reproductive Nutrition Report*. 2005:5;6–7.

Web Resources

American Association of Clinical Endocrinologists
http://www.aace.com

American Dietetic Association
http://www.eatright.org

American Obesity Association
http://www.obesity.org/education/advisor.shtml
An advocacy organization dedicated to changing policy
and perceptions about obesity. Provides information about
obesity and its prevention and treatment.

American Society for Metabolic and Bariatric Surgery
http://www.asbs.org
Provides review of scientific information about morbid
obesity and surgical treatment.

Centers for Disease Control and Prevention
http://www.cdc.gov
Provides information about obesity, and offers many tips
about healthful eating and exercise.

International Federation for the Surgery of Obesity
http://www.obesity-online.com/ifso

Mayo Clinic
http://www.mayoclinic.com
Provides information about obesity and gastric bypass
surgery.

National Heart, Lung, and Blood Institute
http://www.nhlbi.nih.gov/guidelines
For information on gastric bypass surgery, click Treatment
Guidelines, then Management of Weight Loss, then Strategies, and then Surgery.

**National Institute of Diabetes and Digestive
and Kidney Diseases**
http://www.niddk.nih.gov
Provides information about obesity, weight loss, nutrition,
and gastric bypass surgery.

Obesity Action Coalition
http://obesityaction.org

The Obesity Society
http://www.naaso.org

WebMD
http://www.webmd.com
Provides general information about obesity, nutrition, and
weight-loss options. Lists scientific references.

Weight Management Dietetic Practice Group
http://www.wmdpg.org

Roux-en-Y Gastric Bypass Diet Stages

Note: There is no evidence supporting a specific diet transition. Expert opinion suggests (*a*) a staged approach; (*b*) diet advanced as tolerated.

Diet Stage/Timing	Fluids/Foods Allowed	Guidelines for Clients
Stage I • Days 1 and 2 following surgery	• GBP clear liquids[a], water, ice chips	• If you have a gastrogaffin swallow test for leak, begin sipping liquids after test. • If you are not tested, you may begin diet immediately after surgery.
Stage II • Begin on Day 3 after surgery • Begin multivitamin and mineral supplementation[c] • Priority on hydration and protein intake (to minimize loss of lean body mass)	• Variety of GBP clear liquids[a] • Sugar-free ice pops • GBP full liquids[b]	• Consume ≥ 48–64 oz/d total fluids: ≥ 24–32 oz GBP clear liquids plus 24–32 oz of any combination of GBP full liquids. • Encourage clients to have salty fluids at home (broth, bouillon) within fluid allowance.
Stage III, Week 1 • Begin on Days 10–14 after surgery	• Increased intake of GBP clear liquids[a] • As tolerated, replace GBP full liquids[b] with soft, moist, diced, ground or pureed protein sources: eggs; ground meats, poultry, soft, moist fish; added gravy, bouillon, or light mayonnaise to moisten; cooked beans; hearty bean soups; cottage cheese; low-fat cheese; continue yogurt.	• Have > 48–64 oz of total liquids daily. • Aim to have protein food choices at 3 to 6 small meals daily; you may only be able to tolerate a couple of tablespoons at each meal/snack. • Do not drink with meals; wait ~30 min after each meal before having beverages.

Diet Stage/Timing	Fluids/Foods Allowed	Guidelines for Clients
Stage III • Advance to Stage III as tolerated. • Rapid weight-loss phase	• Add well-cooked, soft vegetables and soft and/or peeled fruit to meals/snacks. • Tough, stringy foods that can block the stoma (eg, raw celery, asparagus stalks) should be avoided. • Clients should continue to consume protein with some fruit or vegetables at each meal; some people tolerate salads 1 month after surgery. • Starches should be limited to whole grain crackers with protein, potatoes, and/or dry low-sugar cereals moistened with milk.	• Staying hydrated is essential and a priority! • Wait 30 minutes after meals before having liquids. • Always eat protein first. • *Avoid* rice, bread, and pasta until you can comfortably consume 60–80 g protein as well as fruits/vegetables daily.
Stage IV • Advance to Stage IV as hunger increases and more food is tolerated. • Vitamin and mineral supplementation daily	• Healthy, balanced solid food diet with protein, fruits, vegetables, and whole grains	• Your calorie needs will be based on your height, weight, age, and activity level.

Gastric bypass (GBP) clear liquids: Noncarbonated liquids without calories, sugar, or caffeine.
GBP full liquids: protein-rich liquids with < 25 g sugar per serving, such as 1% or nonfat milk mixed with whey or soy protein powder; lactose-free milk or soy milk mixed with soy protein powder; light yogurt; plain yogurt; Greek yogurt.
*See Appendix D for supplementation guidelines.
Reprinted with permission from Sue Cummings, MS, RD.

Laparoscopic Adjustable Gastric Banding (LAGB) Diet Stages and Postadjustment Diet Instructions

LAGB DIET STAGES

Note: There is no evidence supporting a specific diet transition. Expert opinion suggests (*a*) a staged approach; (*b*) diet advanced as tolerated.

Diet Stage/Timing	Fluids/Foods Allowed	Guidelines for Clients
Stage I • Days 1 and 2 after surgery	• LAGB clear liquids[a]	• On the first day after surgery, you may have sips of water and ice chips.
Stage II (discharge diet) • Days 2 and 3 after surgery • Begin supplementation: chewable multivitamin/multimineral supplement with iron, twice daily; also, chewable or liquid calcium citrate with vitamin D	• Variety of LAGB clear liquids[a] • LAGB full liquids[b]	• Have > 64 oz total fluids per day. • Daily fluids should include ≥ 24–32 oz LAGB clear liquids[a] plus 32 oz of any combination of LAGB full liquids[b].
Stage III, Week 1[c] • Start Days 10–14 after surgery • Continue vitamin and mineral supplementation	• Increased LAGB clear liquids[a] (total liquids > 64 oz/d) • As tolerated, replace LAGB full liquids[b] with soft, moist, diced, ground, or pureed protein sources: eggs, ground meats, poultry, soft, moist fish; added gravy, bouillon, light mayonnaise to moisten; cooked beans; hearty bean soups; cottage cheese; low-fat cheese, yogurt.	• Be assured that hunger is common and normal within a week or so of LAGB. • Having protein foods (moist, ground choices) for 3 to 6 small meals daily can help you feel satisfied. • Mindful, slow, eating is essential. • Do not to drink with meals; wait ~30 minutes after each meal before drinking.

(continues next page)

Diet Stage/Timing	Fluids/Foods Allowed	Guidelines for Clients
Stage III • Start 4 weeks after surgery; advance as tolerated during rapid weight-loss phase.	• If protein foods are well tolerated, add well-cooked, soft vegetables and soft and/or peeled fruit. • If client tolerates soft, moist, ground, diced, and/or pureed proteins with small amounts of fruits and vegetables, then whole grain crackers may be added (to be eaten with protein). • Rice, bread, and pasta should be avoided.	• Staying hydrated is essential and a priority! • Have protein at every meal, especially if you feel increased hunger before your initial fill or adjustment. • Very well-cooked vegetables may also help you to feel satisfied.
Stage IV • Advance to Stage IV as hunger increases and more food is tolerated • Continue daily vitamin and mineral supplementation	• Healthy balanced solid food diet consisting of adequate protein, fruits, vegetables and whole grains • Tough, stringy foods that can block the stoma (eg, raw celery, asparagus stalks, steak) should be avoided.	• Your calorie needs are based on height, weight, age, and activity level.

Diet Stage/Timing	Fluids/Foods Allowed	Guidelines for Clients
Post-LAGB Fill/Adjustment[d] • ~ 6 weeks after surgery; then ~ every 6 weeks until satiety is reached	• LABG full liquids[a] (see Stage II) for 2 days after fill • Advance to Stage III. Week 1 guidelines as tolerated and use for 4–5 days; then advance to Stages III and IV.	• When diet is advanced to soft solids, pay special attention to mindful eating and chewing until food is a mushy consistency; if food is not well chewed, it could get stuck above stoma of the band.

[a]LABG clear liquids: Noncarbonated liquids with no calories, sugar, or caffeine.

[b]LABG full liquids: Low-sugar, low-fat, protein-rich liquids such as 1% or nonfat milk mixed with whey or soy protein powder (limit to 20 g protein per serving); lactose-free milk/soy milk mixed with soy protein powder; blended light yogurt; plain yogurt.

[c]See Chapter 4 for sample meal plan.

[d]See postadjustment instructions later in this appendix.

Reprinted with permission from Sue Cummings, MS, RD.

LAGB POSTADJUSTMENT DIET INSTRUCTIONS

After all adjustments, it is important that clients adhere to the following diet.

Week 1

For the first 2 days after adjustment, follow LAGB Stage II diet. For the next 5 days, follow Stage III diet.

- Plan 3 meals/d, plus 1–2 protein snacks and daily supplements. Each meal should include 4–6 Tbsp (2–3 oz) pureed/ground/moist protein.
- Plan 1 serving/d of dairy: cottage cheese, yogurt, sugar-free pudding; or 8 oz of nonfat or 1% milk (or Lactaid/soy milk).
- Each meal should take 20–30 minutes to eat. Chew food thoroughly; food should be mushy or almost like liquid before swallowing.
- Wait 30 minutes after eating to drink.
- If food feels stuck, do not drink or eat anything else; walk around until food releases. (If it does not release within 1 hour, call your surgeon or doctor.)
- Any of the following may make you feel excessively full or cause you to experience nausea and/or vomiting:
  - You ate too much and/or too quickly.
  - You took too large a bite, without chewing thoroughly.
  - Food was too dry.
  - Band is too tight.

Week 2

Follow the Stage IV diet, a well-balanced, healthy foods diet.

- Eat meals slowly.
- Plan 3 meals and, depending on hunger, 1 or 2 snacks per day.
- It can be helpful for you to keep food records. Write down the times of your meals and snacks, the foods you eat, and the amounts eaten. Also keep track of any problems you have, such as vomiting or any other symptoms associated with eating.
- Be sure to stay hydrated.

Reasons to Call Your Surgeon

Call your surgeon if any of the following happen within a week of a band adjustment:

- Temperature higher than 100.5 degrees Fahrenheit
- Nausea and vomiting daily or repeated regurgitation or heartburn
- Inability to swallow saliva or drooling
- Persistent pain in the abdomen or chest
- Redness or swelling at the adjustment site

Reprinted with permission from Sue Cummings, MS, RD.

Post–Weight-Loss Surgery Supplementation

> **Note:** Clients with abnormal pre- or postsurgical nutritional deficiencies should be treated beyond these recommendations.

Encourage clients to purchase vitamin and calcium supplements before they go to the hospital for weight-loss surgery (WLS) and to begin taking them at home when discharged. It is very important to instruct clients to take multivitamins every day. After Roux-en-Y gastric bypass (RYGBP), clients' nutritional status should be monitored every 2 to 3 months in the first 6 months, once in the second 6 months, and annually thereafter. After laparoscopic adjustable gastric banding (LAGB), nutritional status should be monitored annually.

MULTIVITAMIN WITH IRON

Nutrient Recommendations

Vitamin supplements vary. Encourage clients to read labels and ensure that each of the vitamins listed here are contained in the multivitamin they take.

Clients should select a multivitamin supplement with iron that includes at minimum the Dietary Reference Intake (DRI) for the following nutrients:

- Iron: DRI = 8 mg/d for men, 18 mg/d for women

- Thiamin: DRI = 1.2 mg/d for men, 1.1 mg/d for women
- Vitamin B-12: DRI = 2.4 mcg/d
- Folic acid: DRI = 400 mcg/d
- Zinc: DRI = 11 mg/d for men; 8 mg/d for women
- Biotin: DRI = 30 mcg/d
- Vitamin K: DRI = 120 mcg/d for men, 90 mcg/d for women

Product Types and Dosage Recommendations

Time-release supplements are *not* recommended for WLS clients. Liquid vitamins may be better absorbed after RYGBP. For the first month following any type of WLS, all clients should take multivitamins in a chewable or liquid form. Clients who have LAGB should always select chewable or liquid vitamins and minerals.

Clients should take two children's or one to two adult complete multivitamin supplements with iron daily.

Absorption Issues

Iron

In RYGBP, major sites of iron absorption (the duodenum and proximal jejunum) are bypassed. Vitamin C facilitates iron absorption. Phytates, tannins, and antacids inhibit iron absorption. Menstruating women may need to supplement with an additional 40 to 65 mg of elemental iron per day.

Vitamin B-12

Acid is needed to cleave vitamin B-12 from a protein source. While some vitamin B-12 can be passively absorbed, absorption of most vitamin B-12, which occurs in the ileum, relies on intrinsic factor (IF), which is produced in the stomach. The lower stomach and duodenum, where vitamin B-12 attaches to the IF, are bypassed in RYGBP.

CALCIUM WITH VITAMIN D

Daily Requirements

In addition to multivitamins, clients will need to take daily calcium supplements with vitamin D that provide post-WLS requirements The DRI for calcium is 1,000 mg/d for men and premenopausal women, and 1,200 mg/d for postmenopausal women. After WLS, requirements may be higher: men and premenopausal women should take 1,200 mg calcium supplements daily; the calcium supplement recommendation for postmenopausal women is 1,500 mg/d.

The DRI for vitamin D is 200 IU/d for individuals younger than 50 years, 400 IU/d for adults between the ages of 51 and 70, and 600 IU/d for adults older than 70. After WLS, clients require 400 to 600 IU/d from supplements.

Recommended Product Types

Calcium citrate is the best source of supplemental calcium after gastric bypass surgery because it does not require an acidic environment for absorption. The new pouch produces little to no acid.

For the first month after RYGBP, clients should use only liquid or chewable forms of calcium with vitamin D supplements. Liquid calcium may be better absorbed after RYGBP.

Tablet forms of calcium supplements are usually large. Therefore, clients with LAGB may need to consume only liquid or chewable forms; pills can get stuck if swallowed whole.

Absorption Issues

Multivitamin supplements should be taken a couple of hours before or after calcium supplements. It is also important for clients to take calcium supplements in divided doses for better absorption.

In RYGBP, absorption of calcium and vitamin D are decreased because the duodenum and proximal jejunum are bypassed.

VITAMIN B-12

New guidelines recommend that RYGBP clients supplement with 350 mcg vitamin B-12 per day *or* 1,000 mcg intramuscular (IM) vitamin B-12 per month *or* 3,000 mcg IM vitamin B-12 every 6 months.

OTHER SUPPLEMENTS

Some programs recommend that RYGBP clients take an additional daily supplement of 40 to 65 mg elemental iron.

For women of childbearing age, a prenatal vitamin may be recommended.

Biochemical Surveillance After Weight-Loss Surgery

RECOMMENDED SCHEDULE FOR LABORATORY TESTING

After weight-loss surgery (WLS), periodic assessment of a client's laboratory values is recommended. Such assessments can help ensure adequate nutrition care (1,2).

The following laboratory data should be assessed every 3 to 6 months in the first year and then annually (1,2):

- Complete blood count, platelet count
- Electrolytes
- Iron studies, serum ferritin
- Vitamin B-12 status, methylmalonic acid, homocysteine
- Liver function
- Lipid profile
- Serum 25-dihydroxyvitamin D; parathyroid hormone
- Serum thiamin
- Serum folate

Additionally, dual X-ray absorptiometry (DEXA) is recommended every 2 years to monitor bone density, especially in postmenopausal women (1,2).

POST-RYGBP CONSIDERATIONS FOR
SELECTED NUTRIENTS

Clients who have had Roux-en-Y gastric bypass surgery (RYGBP) require periodic laboratory tests to measure adequacy of several nutrients: vitamin D, calcium, vitamin B-12, folic acid, thiamin, vitamin K, and iron. Refer to Boxes E.1-E.7 (3–16).

Box E.1   Vitamin D (Vitamin D 25-OH)

Normal serum range: 30–46.7 mg/dL
Biomarkers
- 1–25-dihydroxyvitamin D is the most accurate measure of vitamin D stores.
- If vitamin D is deficient:
  - Parathyroid hormone (PTH) is elevated.
  - Alkaline phosphate (ALP) is elevated.
  - Serum phosphorous is less than normal values.

Deficiencies
Vitamin D deficiency may be caused by the following:
- Poor absorption
- Poor adherence to supplementation
- Limited exposure to sunlight
- Nephrotic syndrome and renal failure

Deficiency may produce secondary hyperparathyroidism.

Repletion
- Ergocalciferol: 50,000 IU one to three times per week for 6 to 8 weeks.
- Recheck laboratory values in 3 to 6 months. If serum levels are normal, resume baseline postoperative supplements and recheck again in 3 months (3).

Source: Data are from references 3 and 4.

Box E.2   Calcium

Normal serum ranges: Serum calcium, 9–10.5 mg/dL;
ionized calcium, 4.5–5.6 mg/dL

Biomarkers

- Elevated parathyroid hormone (PTH)—leads to release of
  calcium from bone, potentially causing bone loss and risk of
  osteoporosis
- Elevated alkaline phosphate (ALP)
- **Note:** Ionized calcium is independent of albumin levels.

Bone density tests are recommended before weight-loss
surgery and every 2 years in postmenopausal and other clients
at high risk of conditions associated with calcium deficiency,
such as osteoporosis.

Other Considerations

If serum calcium is less than normal value, determine whether
serum albumin is low. (Low albumin will falsely reduce serum
calcium.)

Source: Data are from references 5, 6, and 7.

Box E.3   Vitamin B-12 (Cobalamin)

Normal serum range: 160–950 pg/mL

Biomarkers
- Serum vitamin B-12 (cobalamin)
- Compared with serum cobalamin, serum increases in methylmalonic acid and homocysteine are more sensitive early markers of vitamin B-12 deficiency.

Deficiencies
A clinically significant deficiency in vitamin B-12 can cause the following:
- Macrocytic anemia
- Megaloblastosis of the bone marrow
- Leucopenia
- Thrombocytopenia
- Glossitis
- Neurologic derangement

Pernicious anemia, megaloblastic anemia (folate deficiency), or low serum vitamin B-12 can also be signs of malnutrition. Pernicious anemia may not be evident until vitamin B-12 has been depleted for 6 to 18 months.

Thirty percent of RYGBP clients who take only a multivitamin supplement may be unable to maintain normal levels of plasma B-12 at 1 year postsurgery. After 1 year post-RYGBP, the prevalence of B-12 deficiency seems to increase yearly (9).

Repletion (8,10–12)
- If client has neurologic symptoms of vitamin B-12 deficiency or if serum level of vitamin B-12 is < 100 mcg/dL, provide 1,000 mcg intramuscular (IM) vitamin B-12 per day for 4 weeks, then 1,000 mcg IM monthly for 4 months. Recheck serum values in 3 to 4 months.
- If serum vitamin B-12 level is 100–150 pg/dL provide 1,000 mcg IM monthly. Recheck serum values in 3 to 4 months.
- If serum vitamin B-12 level is 150–250 pg/dL, provide 1,000 mcg/d orally. Recheck serum values in 3 to 4 months.

If serum vitamin B-12 is above the reference range, stop vitamin B-12 supplementation and recheck serum levels in 1 to 2 months (11).

Source: Data are from references 8–12.

Box E.4   Folic Acid

Normal serum range: 11–57 mmol/L

Biomarker: Red blood cell folate

Deficiencies

Folate deficiency is uncommon because folate absorption occurs throughout the entire small bowel. It has been theorized that deficiency is usually due to decreased folic acid intake (12).

Severe deficiency can lead to the following:

- Macrocytic anemia
- Leucopenia
- Thrombocytopenia
- Glossitis
- Megaloblastic marrow

Repletion

- If serum folic acid levels are below normal values, the client should take a supplement with 800 mcg folic acid per day. The Tolerable Upper Intake Level (UL) for folic acid supplementation in men and women is 1,000 mcg/d.
- If red blood cell folate level is below normal value, replete vitamin B-12 and give 1,000 mcg of folate daily for 3 months.

Source: Data are from reference 12.

Box E.5   Thiamin (Vitamin B-1)

Normal serum ranges: Women: 30–160 mcg/dL; men: 30–300 mcg/dL

Biomarker: Serum vitamin B-1

Deficiencies

Severe thiamin deficiency can lead to the following (13,14):
- Beri beri
- Acute neurologic deficits
- Wernicke's encephalopathy

Severe deficiency may be due to severe, intractable vomiting.

Repletion
- Persistent or intractable vomiting, especially in the early postoperative period, should be resolved aggressively to prevent severe complications (15).
- Thiamin deficiency in all clients should be promptly treated with 50 to 100 mg thiamin per day, administered intravenously or intramuscularly; recheck serum levels at 3 months.
- Do not administer carbohydrate/glucose solutions without thiamin, because thiamin is needed in carbohydrate metabolism.

Source: Data are from references 13, 14, and 15.

Box E.6   Vitamin K

Biomarkers
- Prothrombin time (PT) (normal range: 10–13 secs)
- Partial thromboplastin time (PTT) (normal range: 60–70 secs)
- Activated partial thromboplastin time (normal range: 30–40 secs)

Deficiencies
- Overt vitamin K deficiency results in impaired blood clotting, which is usually demonstrated by laboratory tests that measure clotting times.
- Symptoms include easy bruising and bleeding (eg, nosebleeds, bleeding gums, blood in urine, blood in the stool, tarry black stools, or extremely heavy menstrual cycles)

Other Considerations
Individuals taking vitamin K antagonists or anticoagulant drugs and individuals with significant liver damage are at risk of deficiency.

Box E.7 Iron

After RYGBP, reduced intake of heme iron, reduced conversion of iron from the ferric to ferrous state, and reduced absorption can all contribute to low serum iron levels, especially in premenopausal women (10).

Normal serum ranges: women: 60–160 mcg/dL; men: 30–300 mcg/dL

Biomarkers
- Total iron-binding capacity (TIBC): measures all protein available to bind mobile iron (normal range: 228–428 mcg/dL)
- Serum ferritin: measure of stored iron (normal range for women: 10–150 ng/m; normal range for men: 12–300 ng/m)

Deficiency
- Low serum levels of iron and ferritin with an elevated TIBC may indicate iron-deficiency anemia.
- Iron deficiency after Roux-en-Y gastric bypass (RYGBP) is most common in menstruating women.
- Recommendations include:
  - Oral supplementation with two 325-mg ferrous sulfate tablets daily (65 mg elemental iron per tablet) after RYGBP to prevent the development of iron deficiency (10)
  - Oral supplementation with 325 mg iron sulfate plus 250 mg vitamin C daily; increased to three times daily as tolerated if iron saturation is < 10% (8)

Repletion
- Provide 180 to 220 mg of elemental iron daily (16).
- If client's iron saturation is < 10% and serum ferritin level < 10 ng/mL, or if iron saturation is < 7% (regardless of ferritin level), then provide 325 mg iron sulfate and 250 mg vitamin C supplements daily. Increase supplements to three times daily as tolerated (8).
- Intravenous iron dextran or iron sucrose is used regularly; many clients require intravenous iron several times a year.

Data are from references 8, 10, and 16.

REFERENCES

1. Mechanick JI, Kushner RF, Sugerman HJ, for the writing group. Executive summary of the recommendations of the American Association of Clinical Endocrinologists, the Obesity Society, and the American Society for Metabolic and Bariatric Surgery medical guidelines for clinical practice for the perioperative nutritional, metabolic and nonsurgical support of the bariatric surgery patient. *Endocrin Pract.* 2008;14:318–336.

2. Saltzman E, Anderson W, Apovian CM, Cummings S, et al. Criteria for patient selection and multidisciplinary evaluation and treatment of the weight loss surgery patient. *Obes Res.* 2005;13: 234–243.

3. Goode LR, Brolin RE, Chowdhury HA, Shapses SA. Bone and gastric bypass surgery: effects of dietary calcium and vitamin D. *Obes Res.* 2004;12:40–47.

4. Clements RH, Katasani VG, Palepu R, et al. Incidence of vitamin deficiency after laparoscopic Roux-en-Y gastric bypass in a university hospital setting. *Am Surg.* 2006;72:1196–1202.

5. Shah M, Simha V, Garg A. Review: long-term impact of bariatric surgery on body weight, comorbidities and nutritional status. *J Clin Endocrinol Metab.* 2006;91:4223–4321.

6. Bloomberg RD, Fleishman A, Nalle JE, Herron DM, Kini S. Nutritional deficiencies following bariatric surgery: what have we learned? *Obes Surg.* 2005;15:145–154.

7. Riedt CS, Brolin RE, Sherrell RM, Field MP, Shapses SA. True fractional calcium absorption is decreased after Roux-en-Y gastric bypass surgery. *Obesity.* 2006;14:1940–1948.

8. Shikora SA, Kim JJ, Tarnoff ME. Nutrition and gastrointestinal complications of bariatric surgery. *Nutr Clin Pract.* 2007;22:29–40.

9. Rhode BM, Arseneau P, Cooper BA, Katz M, Gilfix BM, MacLean LD. Vitamin B-12 deficiency after gastric surgery for obesity. *Am J Clin Nutr.* 1996;63:103–109.

10. Tucker ON, Szomstein S, Rosenthal RJ. Nutritional consequences of weight loss surgery. *Med Clin N Am.* 2007;91:499–514.

11. Halverson JD. Micronutrient deficiencies after gastric bypass for morbid obesity. *Am Surg.* 1986;52:594–598.

12. Elliot K. Nutritional considerations after bariatric surgery. *Crit Care Nurs Q.* 2003;26:133–138.

13. Angstadt JD, Bodziner RA. Peripheral polyneuropathy from thiamin deficiency following laparoscopic Roux-en-Y gastric bypass. *Obes Surg.* 2005;15:890–89.

14. Shuster MH, Vazquez JA. Nutritional concerns related to Roux-en-Y gastric bypass: what every clinician needs to know. *Crit Care Nurs Q.* 2005;28:227–260.

15. Singh S, Kumar A. Wernicki encephalopathy after obesity surgery: a systematic review. *Neurology.* 2007;68:807–811.

16. Fugioka K. Follow-up of nutritional and metabolic problems after bariatric surgery. *Diabetes Care.* 2005;28:481–484.

Education Session Guides and Sample Questionnaires

EDUCATION SESSIONS

The registered dietitian can lead the following client education sessions (Boxes F.1 and F.2) alone or co-lead education sessions with other team members (1–7).

**Box F.1   Sample Outline for Weight-Loss Surgery Information
            Session**

1. Define *obesity*
   a. Medical term
   b. Excess body fat
   c. Estimated by body mass index (BMI)
2. Educate about BMI
   a. Provide chart showing BMI for different heights and weights.
   b. Define overweight and obesity using BMI.
3. Educate regarding indications for weight-loss surgery
   a. National Institutes of Health and National Heart, Lung, and
      Blood Institute criteria
   b. Additional program criteria (program fees, scheduling
      commitments, etc)
4. Contraindications to surgery
   a. End-stage lung disease
   b. Unstable cardiovascular disease
   c. Multi-organ failure
   d. Class C cirrhosis
   e. Gastric varices
   f. Uncontrolled psychiatric disorder
   g. Ongoing substance abuse
   h. Noncompliance with medical regimens; appointments
5. Describe types of surgery
   a. Roux-en-Y gastric bypass (RYGBP)
      i. Small stomach pouch
      ii. Alteration of food pathway
      iii. Causes decreased hunger, increased fullness
      iv. Mean weight loss in first 2 years is ~65% of excess body
          weigh and is typically followed by a regain of about 15%,
          or a 50% excess body weight maintained long-term (1–3).
      v. Most commonly a laparoscopic procedure; may need to be
         converted to open surgery
   b. Complications of RYGBP
      i. Intestinal obstruction, marginal ulcers, constipation,
         gallstones, anastomotic strictures, incisional hernias,
         dumping syndrome
      ii. Risk of vitamin and mineral deficiencies; requires life-long
          supplementation
      iii. Mortality: in-hospital mortality rate is 0.14%; 30-day
           mortality rate is 0.29% (4).

(continues next page)

Box F.1   Sample Outline for Weight-Loss Surgery Information Session *(continued)*

---

    c. Benefits of RYGBP: dramatic improvements in:
        i.   Type 2 diabetes mellitus
        ii. Gastroesophageal reflux
        iii. Hypercholesterolemia
        iv. Obstructive sleep apnea
        v. Hypertension
        vi. Osteoarthritis
        vii. Asthma
    d. Laparoscopic adjustable gastric band (LAGB)
        i.   Small stomach pouch
        ii. Pouch outlet adjustable
        iii. No change in food pathway
        iv. LABG is associated with substantially less excess weight loss than RYGBP at 5 years (2,3).
    e. Complications of LAGB
        i.   Band slippage
        ii. Band erosion
        iii. Band/port site infection
        iv. Intolerance of band
        v. Additional operations to address complications (5,6)
        vi. Mortality rate is 1 in 1,000 (0.1%) (2)
        vii. Requires regular fills (adjustments)
    f. Benefits of LAGB: Less risk than RYGBP (but also fewer benefits); improvements in comorbidities are less dramatic than RYGBP

6. Expectations
    a   Review realistic estimates of short- and long-term weight loss.
    b. Explain that the magnitude and sustainability of weight loss and benefits vary by type of procedure and client characteristics (3,7).
    c. Inform clients of the potential for weight regain

7. Preparing for surgery
    a. Although not recommended, many clients prepare for WLS by going on a last "celebration," eating all of their favorite foods.
    b. Explain that weight-loss surgery is a lifestyle change, and therefore unlike prior experiences with going on and off diets, and that the best way for clients to prepare for surgery is by getting in their best shape, losing weight, weaning from caffeine, getting physically active, and quitting smoking.

Reprinted with permission from Sue Cummings, MS, RD.

Box F.2   Presurgery Nutrition Education Session

Presurgery Guidelines: Setting Expectations, Starting Habits
- Clients are expected to be ambulatory after surgery to avoid blood clots; encourage ambulatory clients to be prepared to take short frequent walks throughout the day.
- Clients should wean themselves from caffeine to avoid immediate withdrawal symptoms after surgery (caffeine should be avoided during the first days of recovery to prevent dehydration).
- Clients should wean themselves from carbonated and sweetened beverages.
- Clients should practice mindful eating.

Diet Stages: Postoperative Diet Based on Nutritional Needs
- In the first days and weeks after surgery, emphasis is on hydration and adequate protein intake; texture; and slow, mindful eating and chewing.
- The amount of food clients can eat, the pace at which they can eat, and the types of foods they can tolerate is a function of healing; the pace at which the diet is advanced will depend on what the individual client can tolerate.

Diet Stage I
- Hospital stay for a Roux-en-Y gastric bypass (RYGBP) client without complications is usually two nights.
- Some centers discharge laparoscopic gastric band (LAGB) clients on the day of surgery, others have clients stay one night.
- The inpatient diet protocol should be part of the presurgical client education materials.

Diet Stage II
- Clients are discharged with diet orders to advance to stage II (RYGBP or LAGB clear and full liquids) at home.
- The health care team should provide printed materials including a shopping list, guidelines for hydration and sample meal plans, and blank records for recording total intake.
- Clients should have a schedule of postoperative visits, including an appointment with the registered dietitian (RD) two weeks after surgery.

(continues next page)

Box F.2   Presurgery Nutrition Education Session *(continued)*

Education Materials
- Surgical centers have different protocols for distributing client education materials before surgery. Some provide all the diet stages (see Appendixes B and C) before surgery. Others provide education for the first two diet stages and have clients schedule an appointment with the RD to advance to other stages; this is to discourage clients from advancing on their own without adequate instruction.
- Additional education materials include the following:
  - Fact sheets on vitamin and minerals and supplements: vitamin B-12, folate, vitamin D, iron, calcium, and vitamin K
  - List and schedule of laboratory tests to monitor nutritional adequacies
  - List of medications to avoid, including those that may put clients at high risk of developing ulcers
  - Fact sheet on lactose intolerance
  - Fact sheet on recognizing signs and symptoms of dehydration

---

Source: Reprinted with permission from Sue Cummings, MS, RD.

SAMPLE CLIENT QUESTIONNAIRES

Figures F.1 through F.4 are examples of questionnaires that might be used in nutrition assessment and intervention with weight-loss surgery clients.

**Figure F.1 Questionnaire for First Nutrition Visit
After RYGBP**

Today's date: _____ Date of surgery: _____

Today's weight: _____

1. Did you have complications after weight-loss surgery that affected your ability to follow the diet guidelines you were given?　　No　　Yes

2. If yes, explain:

    _____

3. List any medications you are currently taking:

    _____

4. Check any of the following that you are experiencing:
    ☐ Nausea episodes　　☐ Vomiting episodes
    ☐ Dumping syndrome　　☐ Diarrhea
    ☐ Constipation

5. For each box checked in Question 4, please list the triggers or causes:_____

6. Have you been consuming at least 24 oz of "**full**" liquid every day?　　No　　Yes

7. If you are not able to consume 24 oz, how much are you consuming? _____

8. Check the liquids you are consuming:
    ☐ Protein powder mixed with milk
    ☐ Instant breakfast mixed with milk
    ☐ Light blended or plain yogurt
    ☐ Tomato soup with milk
    ☐ Milk alone
    ☐ Sugar-free pudding
    ☐ Other _____

9. Have you been consuming at least 24 oz "**clear**" liquid every day?　　No　　Yes

---

(continues next page)

**Figure F.1   Questionnaire for First Nutrition Visit
After RYGBP** *(continued)*

---

10. Check the liquids you are consuming:
    ☐ Water ☐ Other sugar-free clear liquids
    ☐ Sugar-free ice pops ☐ Other (list)

11. Have you started taking a multivitamin?
    No   Yes (list type) _____

12. Have you started taking a calcium supplement?
    No   Yes (list type) _____

13. How many short walks (5–10 minutes) do you take each
    day? _____

14. Do you have a schedule of all of your nutrition follow-up
    groups or appointments?   Yes   No

Client should sign and print name clearly below questionnaire.

Reprinted with permission from Sue Cummings, MS, RD.

Figure F.2   Questionnaire for Post–Weight-Loss Surgery Nutrition Visit, Diet Stages III and IV

Today's date: _____ Date of surgery: _____

Who is your surgeon? _____

Which procedure did you have? (circle one)
Gastric bypass   Gastric band

Today's weight: _____

Total weight loss since surgery: _____

1. Check any of the following that you are experiencing:
   ☐ Nausea episodes   ☐ Vomiting episodes
   ☐ Dumping syndrome (after eating, you have one or more of the following symptoms: flushing, sweatiness, rapid heartbeat, dizziness, cramping)
   ☐ Diarrhea   ☐ Constipation
   ☐ Food gets stuck   ☐ Excessive fatigue
   ☐ Dizziness, especially when going from sitting to standing

2. For each box checked in Question 1, please list the triggers or causes:
   _____

3. Other symptoms/complaints:
   _____

4. Please write down what you eat and drink on a typical day (approximate times that you eat, foods/amounts, fluids/amounts): _____

5. Do you have protein at most meals or snacks?
   No   Yes

6. Do you drink liquids with meals?
   No   Yes   (amount: _____)

7. Do you drink carbonated beverages?
   No   Yes   (amount: _____)

(continues next page)

**Figure F.2   Questionnaire for Post–Weight-Loss Surgery
Nutrition Visit, Diet Stages III and IV *(continued)***

---

8. Do you drink alcohol?
   No   Yes   (amount: _____)

9. How many ounces of clear liquids do you drink in a day?

   _____

10. Are you taking a multivitamin with minerals and iron
    daily?
    No   Yes   (list type) _____

11. Are you taking a calcium supplement daily?
    No   Yes   (list type) _____

12. List other vitamins or supplements that you take:

    _____

13. Check the answers that describe you:
    ☐ I never get hungry.
    ☐ I get hungry sometimes.
    ☐ I am hungry throughout the day.
    ☐ I plan and prepare all of my meals and make time to sit
       and eat mindfully.
    ☐ I practice eating slowly.

13. List foods and beverages that your body does *not* tolerate:

    _____

14. Do you exercise regularly?
    No   Yes   (list types of activity)

15. How many days a week do you exercise? _____
    How many minutes per session? _____
    Per day? _____ Per week? _____

16. Are you having difficulty adjusting to your diet?
    No   Yes   (please explain) _____

17. Do you need additional psychology or dietitian visits?
    No   Yes

Client should sign and print name clearly below questionnaire.

Reprinted with permission from Sue Cummings, MS, RD.

Figure F.3   LAGB Hunger Survey (used to determine whether "fill" is needed)

Today's date: _____ Today's weight: _____

Date of last fill: _____ Weight at last fill: _____

The following questions ask about experiences with hunger and fullness. Your feelings may vary from day to day or from meal to meal. Answer questions about how you feel "on average."

Hunger
In the following questions, hunger is defined as a physical feeling in the body.

1. Check all that describe your feelings of hunger.
   - ☐ Feeling of emptiness in your body
   - ☐ Fatigue
   - ☐ General feeling of needing to eat or drink
   - ☐ Physical sensations in your stomach (such as grumbling or discomfort)
   - ☐ Abdominal pain   ☐ Light-headedness
   - ☐ Irritability   ☐ Other: _____
   - ☐ I don't know what hunger feels like.
   - ☐ I never experience hunger.

2. Since your last *fill,* how often have you experienced hunger?
   - ☐ Never   ☐ Every few days
   - ☐ Almost every day   ☐ 1–2 times a day
   - ☐ Several times a day   ☐ Always hungry

3. Since your last *fill,* how strong have your feelings of hunger typically been?
   - ☐ Unable to eat   ☐ Not hungry
   - ☐ Slightly hungry   ☐ Moderately hungry
   - ☐ Very hungry   ☐ Absolutely "starving"

(continues next page)

Figure F.3   LAGB Hunger Survey (used to determine whether "fill" is needed) *(continued)*

Fullness

The following questions address feelings of fullness. These feelings may include a general *physical* feeling that you have had enough to eat.

4. Since your last *fill,* how full do you feel, in general, after you finish a snack or meal?

   ☐ Totally empty   ☐ Not at all full
   ☐ Slightly full   ☐ Moderately full
   ☐ Very full   ☐ Absolutely "stuffed"

5. Since your last *fill*, how long after you start eating do you typically notice feelings of fullness?

   ☐ 0–5 minutes   ☐ 6–10 minutes
   ☐ 11–15 minutes   ☐ 16–20 minutes
   ☐ 20–30 minutes   ☐ More than 30 minutes

6. Since your last *fill*, how long after feeling full do you generally become physically hungry again?

   ☐ 0–14 minutes   ☐ 15–30 minutes
   ☐ 30 minutes–1 hour   ☐ 1–3 hours
   ☐ More than 3 hours   ☐ I never feel hungry

Reprinted with permission from Sue Cummings, MS, RD.

Figure F.4 Nutrition Assessment Questionnaire for Postsurgical Clients in Maintenance Phase

Today's date: _____ Date of surgery: _____

Who is your surgeon? _____

Which procedure did you have?

      (circle one) Gastric bypass Gastric band

Today's weight: _____ Total weight loss since surgery: _____

Height (in/cm): _____

1. List illnesses or medical conditions diagnosed before weight-loss surgery: _____

2. List medications taken before weight-loss surgery: _____

3. List current illnesses or medical conditions: _____

4. List medications currently taken: _____

5. Please write down what you eat and drink on a typical day (approximate times, foods/amounts, fluids/amounts): _____

6. Do you have a protein food at most meals or snacks?
   No   Yes

7. Do you drink liquids with meals?
   No   Yes (list amount) _____

8. Do you drink carbonated beverages?
   No   Yes (list amount) _____

9. Do you drink alcohol?
   No   Yes (list amount) _____

10. Are you taking a multivitamin with minerals/iron daily?
    No   Yes (list type) _____

11. Are you taking a calcium supplement daily?
    No   Yes (list type) _____

12. List other vitamins or supplements that you take: _____

13. List foods/beverages that your body does *not* tolerate: _____

(continues next page)

Figure F.4   Nutrition Assessment Questionnaire for Postsurgical Clients in Maintenance Phase *(continued)*

---

14. Do you exercise regularly? No Yes (list types of activity)
    _____

15. How many days a week do you exercise? _____
    How many minutes per session? _____
    Per day? _____ Per week? _____

16. Average number of steps taken per day: _____

17. Are you having difficulty adjusting to diet and healthy
    lifestyle changes?   No Yes (explain) _____

* * * * * *

RD Assessment

% excess body weight loss:_____ BMI: _____

Estimated energy expenditure
    (use Mifflin-St. Jeor equation): _____

Men: RMR =
    $(9.99 \times Wt [kg]) + (6.25 \times Ht [cm]) - (4.02 \times Age[y]) + 5$

Women RMR =
    $(9.99 \times Wt [kg]) + (6.25 \times Ht [cm]) - (4.92 \times Age [y]) - 161$

Activities of daily living (circle one):
        Sedentary   Moderate   Very active

Laboratory Data

☐ Per Client   ☐ Per Report

Date:_____

Glucose: _____ HbA1C: _____

Vitamin D: _____ PTH: _____ Vitamin B-12: _____

Iron: _____ Ferritin: _____ TIBC: _____

Calcium: _____ Hb/Hct : _____

TG: _____ LDL: ____ HDL: _____

Nutrition Diagnosis: _____

PES Statement:_____

Nutrition Prescription: _____

Nutrition Intervention plan/goal(s): _____

Registered dietitian's signature/contact information

Reprinted with permission from Sue Cummings, MS, RD.

REFERENCES

1. Pories WJ, Swanson MS, MacDonald KG, et al. Who would have thought it? An operation proves to be the most effective therapy for adult-onset diabetes mellitus. *Ann Surg*. 1995;222:339–250.

2. Angrisani L, Lorenzo M, Borrelli V. Laparoscopic adjustable gastric banding versus Roux-en-Y gastric bypass: 5 year results of a prospective randomized trial. *Surg Obes Relat Dis*. 2007;3:127–134.

3. Sjostrom L, Lindroos AK, Peltonen M, et al. Lifestyle, diabetes and cardiovascular risk factors 10 years after bariatric surgery. *N Eng J Med*. 2004;351:2683–2693.

4. Pratt GM, Mclees B, Pories WJ. The ASBS Bariatric Surgery Centers of Excellence program: a blueprint for quality improvement. *Surg Obes Relat Dis*. 2006;2:497–503.

5. O'Brien PE, Dixon JB, Laurie C, et al. Treatment of mild to moderate obesity with laparoscopic adjustable gastric banding or an intensive medical program: a randomized trial. *Ann Intern Med*. 2006;144:625–633.

6. Fried M, Peskova M. Gastric banding: advantages and complications. A 5-year and 10-year follow-up. *Obes surg*. 1995;5:372–374.

7. Maggard MA, Shugarman LR, Suttorp M, et al. Meta-analysis: surgical treatment of obesity. *Ann Intern Med*. 2005;142:547–559.

appendix g

Complications

COMPLICATIONS OF LAPAROSCOPIC ADJUSTABLE GASTRIC BANDING (LAGB) (1,2)

Band Erosion

- Band will erode through the stomach wall; erosion rarely leads to free perforation or sepsis.
- Etiology is unclear, but thought to be due to operative injury to the gastric wall or band that is too tight and overinflated.
- Band erosion is best diagnosed by endoscopy and treated by band removal.

Esophageal Dilatation

- This is a serious condition, with a risk of esophageal motility dysfunction.
- The etiology is likely to be overinflation of the band.
- Esophageal dilatation may lead to back-up of consumed food in the distal esophagus.
- Condition is diagnosed by fluoroscopic X-ray of upper gastrointestinal tract.
- Condition may be asymptomatic; yearly testing is suggested.
- Esophageal dilatation may require band removal.

Band Prolapse

- Prolapse results in obstruction of pouch or herniation of fundus.
- Etiology is unknown but may be poor fixation or dietary noncompliance.
- Band prolapse is diagnosed by fluoroscopic x-ray of upper gastrointestinal tract.
- Condition may resolve with band deflation.
- Signs and symptoms of prolapse include abdominal pain, nausea/vomiting, gastroesophageal reflux, dysphagia (difficulty swallowing liquids), gastric obstruction.
- Treatment for prolapse involves the following:
  - Saline removal to increase the stoma
  - Diet texture regression to liquids and then soft foods
  - Allowing the stomach to slip back down
  - Review of eating style changes
  - New operation to secure the band

LONG-TERM NUTRITIONAL DEFICIENCIES
POST–ROUX-EN-Y GASTRIC BYPASS

Nutrient	Causes of Deficiency
Iron	• Malabsorption due to the bypass of duodenum and proximal jejunum • Intolerance of iron-rich red meat • Reduced production of hydrochloric acid, which is required to reduce ferric iron to ferrous state for absorption
Vitamin B-12	• Achlorhydria preventing cleavage from food • Decreased tolerance of milk and meat • Poor secretion of intrinsic factor
Folate	• Decreased intake
25-hydroxy vitamin D	• Obese clients with presurgery deficiency are at higher risk for vitamin D deficiency than nonobese individuals. • Lack of sun exposure; use of sunscreen
Calcium	• Malabsorption, bypass of the duodenum and proximal jejunum • Intolerance of lactose, leading to restricted intake of food sources of calcium without supplementation • Serum calcium maintained by release of calcium from bone
Vitamin A	• Vitamin A absorption may be limited due to the short common channel and delayed mixing of fat with pancreatic enzymes and bile salts as a result of bypassing the duodenum.

Source: Data are from references 1–4.

REFERENCES

1. Shikora SA, Kim JJ, Tarnoff ME. Nutrition and gastrointestinal complications of bariatric surgery. *Nutr Clin Pract*. 2007;22:29–40.

2. Clements RH, Katasani VG, Palepu R, et al. Incidence of vitamin deficiency after laparoscopic Roux-en-Y gastric bypass in a university hospital setting, *Am Surg*. 2006;72:1196–1202.

3. Shah M, Simha V, Garg A. Review: long-term impact of bariatric surgery on body weight, comorbidities and nutritional status. *J Clin Endocrinol Metab*. 2006;91:4223–4321.

4. Bloomberg RD, Fleishman A, Nalle JE, Herron DM, Kini S. Nutritional deficiencies following bariatric surgery: what have we learned? *Obes Surg*. 2005;15:145–154.

appendix h

Binge Eating Disorder Diagnostic Criteria

Criterion	Description
A	Recurrent episodes of binge eating, characterized by both of the following: 1. Eating in a discrete period of time, an amount of food that is definitely larger than most people would eat during a similar period of time and under similar circumstances 2. A sense of lack of control over eating during the episode (e.g., a feeling that one cannot stop eating or control what or how much one is eating)
B	The binge-eating episodes are associated with 3 (or more) of the following: 1. Eating much more rapidly than normal 2. Eating until feeling uncomfortably full 3. Eating large amounts of food when not feeling physically hungry 4. Eating alone because of being embarrassed by how much one is eating 5. Feeling disgusted with oneself, depressed, or very guilty after overeating
C	Marked distress regarding binge eating is present.
D	The binge eating occurs, on average, at least 2 days a week for 6 months.
E	The binge is not associated with regular use of inappropriate compensatory behaviors (eg, purging, fasting, excessive exercise) and does not occur exclusively during the course of anorexia nervosa or bulimia nervosa.

Reproduced with permission from the *Diagnostic and Statistical Manual of Mental Disorders, Text Revision, Fourth Edition* (Copyright 2000). American Psychiatric Association.

index

Page number followed by *b* indicates box; *f,* figure; *t,* table.